ARTHRITIS:

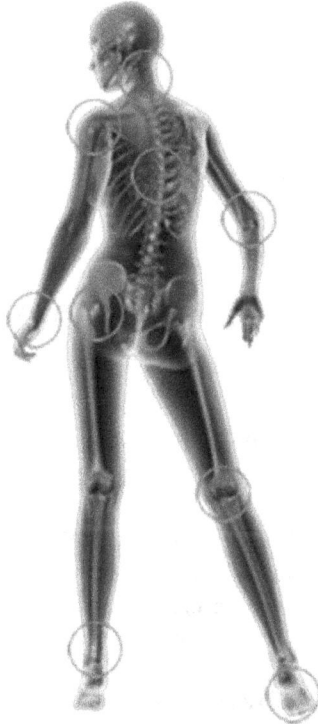

To Conquer It
Check for These Cause(s)

Pamela Levin, R.N.

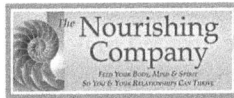

The Nourishing Company
FEED YOUR BODY, MIND & SPIRIT
SO YOU & YOUR RELATIONSHIPS CAN THRIVE

Published by The Nourishing Company
www.nourishingcompany.com

Library of Congress Cataloging-in-Publication Data
Levin, Pamela
Arthritis: To Conquer it Address the Cause(s)
ISBN-13: 978-0-9672718-5-9
ISBN-10-0967271851

1. Health 2. Arthritis 3. Alternative Medicine 4.Title

Cover and book design by Jerri Jo Idarius, Creation Designs
www.creation-designs.com

The information in this book is for educational purposes only. It is not
intended to diagnose or prescribe for medical or psychological
conditions, nor to prevent, treat, mitigate or cure such conditions. A
one-to-one relationship with a qualified health care professional
cannot be replaced by this written material and does not take the place
of medical advice.

As a reader, you are encouraged to use it as a resource to make your
health care decisions in partnership with a qualified health care
professional. Ultimately, if you choose to do anything based on what
you read or hear, you and you alone are responsible.

TABLE OF CONTENTS

ACKNOWLEDGMENTS

Many thanks to the health practitioners and researchers who searched beyond symptoms to discover causes and the effective protocols to address them.

Also to those who developed systems for delivering that information to other practitioners and clients.

My personal mentor list for the material in this book includes:

*Lee Vagt, D.C.,his system of Neurointegration;
*D.A.Versendaal, D.C., his system of Contact Reflex Analysis;
*Freddie Ulan, D.C., his system of Nutrition Response Testing;
*Frank Springob, D.C., his system of Morphogenetic Field Testing;
*phytotherapists Kerry Bone MCPP FNHAA FNIMH DipPhyto Bsc(Hons), founder of MediHerb of Australia
*Lee Carroll, BHSC, also of MediHerb
*Eric Berne, MD, founder of Transactional Analysis.

Ongoing gratitude to those who continue to educate me, especially Kim Sperry, ACN; Don Lawson of the Working Body, Oakland, Ca.; Kerry Bone, Founder of MediHerb Australia; and Linda Ryan, ND (Aus), AHG Registered Herbalist.

Also to readers of the manuscript for your many helpful comments which were pivotal in the final form of this material, especially: Beverley Spence, Leslie Lind and Don Macken.

Pamela Levin, R.N.

INTRODUCTION

You can't avoid pain in life;
it's how you handle pain that defines you.

Joint pains are not just uncomfortable. They can also set you up with nagging, constant worries. "Am I falling apart?" "What if I can't work?" "What if I can't take care of my kids?" "Or even take care of myself?" "Is it going to get worse?" "What if I have to endure a lot of pain?" " Is this the beginning of the end?"

Before you know it, you see yourself wasting away in some dark hospital corner, or being carried out your own front door feet first. So of course, you want them to go away as quickly as possible. That's why it's so important to understand what joint symptoms are. Simply put:

Joint ***symptoms*** are indications of ***something else.***

Think of them like the warning lights in your car that give you a 'heads up' about something else - low oil, a door not shut tight, a seat belt not engaged, and so on. What would happen if you dealt with that warning light by disconnecting the light? Symptom gone, right? Oops. Using this approach, you're going to be really sorry down the line, and it's going to cost you a LOT of money.

The same is true when you suppress your joint pain with medications. You've basically disconnected your body's equivalent of that early warning light. If you think your arthritic *symptoms* are the problem, so you just make them go away, you are asking for trouble. Why? Because:

Symptoms are NOT causes.

One symptom - in this case, joint inflammation - can be produced by a variety of causes just as car warning lights can indicate a variety of problems. Each requires a different action to fix them. The same is true when your body/mind makes a warning light in the form of joint inflammation symptoms.

That variety of causes and what you can do about them is the subject of this book, and is the first essential distinction about the approach detailed here: its pages present some top causes at the root of joint inflammation symptoms. To underscore the point:

To resolve a symptom, you will need to
address the cause.

Taking this approach, you and your health care team can become detectives, tracking down your body's message until you get it correctly translated and addressed. That is true resolution. Now, you're not merely squashing the symptom while below the surface its actions continue unabated. Instead, you become free of it, plus you've also improved your overall health. Also, you may well have prevented a major health disaster down the line. (i-1)

Imagine the difference that approach could make if it were applied not just by you, but also by the over 50 million adults with doctor-diagnosed arthritis. What if the 1 in 4 people over age 18, who experience this number one cause of disability in the nation actually addressed the root of their symptoms effectively? What would happen to the more than $156 billion lost annually in wages and medical expenses? What would happen to medical costs if the more than 100 million outpatient visits and an estimated 6.7 million hospitalizations due to arthritis were massively decreased and the repeat visits and prescriptions eliminated?

And how would the individual lives and families affected by the significant functional limitations of arthritis sufferers change? - the one in six who are unable to walk even ¼ mile, the one in 22 who have trouble grasping an object, the one in nine who can't climb stairs. And the one in 250 developing children who also have arthritis. The effects of addressing it effectively would be felt across all the ages, races and genders who suffer from it. All the more reasons to heed that bodily 'warning light', get to the root of the problem and resolve it. (i-2)

The second essential difference in this approach is about how to deal with causes once they're identified. If you were to answer the question, 'What is the human body made of?" you would have to arrive at one answer, "Food!" This means that in order to give your body what it needs to resolve any health issues, it will require the proper food.

The body can't make or repair living tissues out of dead material – instead it requires the living substances contained in food. To address causes of joint inflammation and repair those specific tissues, it requires _specific live foods_. Using such live foods concentrated to clinical potency is the basis for clinical nutrition and is a foundation of actually being able to resolve joint inflammation and repair tissues.

The third and last essential difference about the approach detailed here has to do with the use of organic herbs. Specific plants hold the power to direct and support resolving the causes that give rise to arthritis symptoms. As you no doubt recognize, plants are living vegetation that, unlike their animal relatives, are rooted to one place. They can't run or hide or attack to protect themselves if some animal wants to eat them. Instead, they defend themselves through making specific chemical substances.

Plants have had some 700 million years to create the adaptations they need to survive and reproduce. They may create a substance that makes them smell bad or taste bad so a hungry animal passes them by or even gets poisoned if it takes a bite. They may generate other ones to protect themselves against fungi or viruses. This ability allows them to survive and reproduce in the same location as the insects and animals that want to eat them.

And if they're being munched on, they can "even release powerful airborne chemicals that attract a variety of larger predators, such as wasps, dragonflies or even small mammals and lizards. These animals are drawn to the plant being eaten, where it can make quick work of the irritating insects doing the damage." (i-3)

All these plant cells protections are good news for us. The proteins they generate to protect themselves have medicinal properties that can help us heal and regenerate. What this means for joint inflammation and pain, is that we can use certain of these nature-made plant chemicals to address their causes.

Now that you know these three essential differences: determining causes, providing the right living whole foods concentrated to clinical potency and using the medicinal properties of whole organic herbs, you're ready for the specifics.

Before we get to these – a few pointers. First, you're likely to be tempted into the same mistake health professionals make who are beginning their training, which is to think you have all the conditions outlined here. As a word of assurance: that is _very_ unlikely. Many people have one major contributor, while some have one or two minor ones also.

Use your time with this material to make notes about what you want to find out from your health practitioner and leave the diagnosis to the professionals. There is competent help out there. In fact, the entire last chapter is devoted to finding exactly the help you need.

So take a deep breath, and use this material to inform yourself about the possibilities. Then if you need to, find a competent professional you feel good about working with, and let them do their job. It's not up to you to diagnose your own condition – or to treat it on your own.
Second, a note about the content of each subject. To be effective in dealing with each condition, you have to start by understanding it. Therefore you'll find that each topic begins with an explanation about what's going on – the dynamics that result in arthritis. This is followed by a section about what you can do. Further, as some readers want technical information to back up broader statements while others find it distracting, look for this greater detail in the endnotes for each chapter.

Third, once you've completed the first two chapters, you can read the subjects in any order you like. You'll likely find subjects you feel more drawn to than others, so feel free to read in the order in which you're inspired to do.

Fourth since arthritis causes pain which causes emotional stress, be sure to include the chapter on Emotional Stress as soon as you're ready.

Last, as you read you will find some overlap in symptoms with different causes. You'll find that easy to understand if you remember that the body responds to most invaders and injury with inflammation and heat, among other reactions. Again, you'll find that difficult to sort out for yourself, so seek help. To underscore the message: resources are listed at the end of the book.

The point is, there are avenues of inquiry that can lead to successful resolution of your arthritis symptoms. Sometimes you just have to step out of your conditioned way of thinking to find them. It's hoped that the rest of this book serves that function.
That said, let's get to it!

***

Endnotes:

(i-1) <u>Symptoms - The Best Place to Start Resolving Them</u>
http://www.betterhealthbytes.com/Volume-3-Issue-51.html.

(i-2) from The Arthritis Foundation
http://www.arthritis.org/about-arthritis/understanding-arthritis/arthritis-statistics-facts.php.

(i-3) https://www.scienceabc.com/nature/how-do-plants-defend-themselves-dangers-attacks.html

1. WHAT IS ARTHRITIS?

"We cannot change what we are not aware of, and once we are aware, we cannot help but change."
— Sheryl Sandberg (COO of Facebook)

I t's a scene repeated countless times, not that you wanted to be one of those numbers. It starts when you have pain in a joint. You notice it gets worse if the temperature or barometric pressure drops.

You go to the doctor and say, "Doc, I've got inflammation in my joint(s) and it really hurts. What's going on?"
You go through some expensive tests and the answer comes back: "You've got arthritis." When your pain is given this label, what have you learned? Only one thing: the Latin name for joint inflammation.

The word itself is derived from two ancient languages: the first part comes from the Greek prefix 'arth' meaning 'joint' and the suffix '-itis' which means 'inflammation of'. Together they refer to inflammation of a joint or joints.

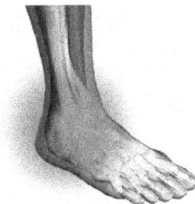

Figure 1This joint is inflamed and painful

Simply put, arthritis is a *symptom*. You start to question if you have it when you feel pain in a joint. However, arthritis is *only* a symptom, and it is one that has many causes. Therefore if you want to address it effectively, meaning to eliminate it, you'll need to find and address the cause (or causes.)

That's the purpose of this book – to give you an overview of the most common actual causes of this symptom, and to summarize ways to address them.

Now that you have a working arthritis definition, let's focus next on what kind. That will give you some ideas about what a medical diagnosis of arthritis actually means. It may also hold the keys for you to unlock how to deal with it.

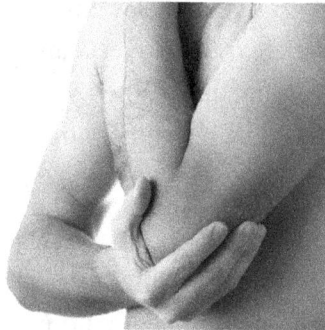

**Figure 2 This man may have played
a few too many tennis games.**

Western medicine uses two main categories for two main types of arthritis - infectious arthritis, also called rheumatoid arthritis, and non-infectious arthritis .

Infectious Arthritis: This refers inflammation of a joint caused by any one or more infectious agents such as bacteria, viruses, parasites, or spirochetes. Some of the more common ones are: gonococcal, pneumococcal, tubercular, staph, strep (which is the infectious agent in rheumatic fever) and in more recent years, Lyme's, a spirochete. Each of these causes will be addressed individually later on, but for now, let's answer the most pressing question people have when they are told they have an infection in a joint, which is, "Is arthritis infectious?"

The answer is no, not technically, because arthritis only means inflammation of the joint. However, the infectious agent may be transmittable, as it is in the case of gonorrhea, strep, staph or tuberculosis.

Knowing that your joint cartilage is being gobbled up or worn away by some such bug, you're armed with knowledge you can use to choose a strategy that invites those bugs to live elsewhere. Then when they do, you can move to the second phase of your strategy, which involves repairing the damage.

Non-Infectious Arthritis: This term refers to all the other causes of joint inflammation. For example 'traumatic arthritis' is the result of sudden or repeated stress on the joint, as in tennis elbow, while 'post-traumatic arthritis' is the result of an injury such as a bump or blow. 'Septic arthritis' is joint inflammation that results from toxicity of some kind - perhaps a food intolerance, heavy metals or pesticides, for example.

Last, there are three types of joint tissue that can become inflamed from any of the above. One type is the bone itself, and this is called 'osteoarthritis'. The second is the joint cartilage itself. To answer what cartilage is, think of the gristle in a piece of meat - that's cartilage. It's a type of very dense, firm and compact connective tissue that's capable of withstanding considerable pressure or tension. Third, the synovial membrane over the joint, and the fluid it contains which lubricates the joint can also become inflamed.

Hip Joint

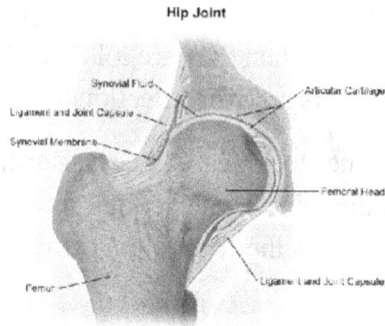

**Figure 3 Basic anatomy of the hip joint,
a common site for joint inflammation.**

To review: no matter which type of joint tissue becomes inflamed, the condition is still referred to as 'arthritis' because some part of the joint is inflamed.

The most important point to remember is that a medical diagnosis of 'arthritis' refers to a _symptom_ and not a cause. If you want to eliminate, instead of merely control or suppress this symptom, you will need to find and effectively address the cause.

And don't worry – you won't have to do it alone. Just read on to start educating yourself about the various possibilities. That way you can match each one of these factors with its relevance based on your own unique history that only you know best. Then you'll be in the perfect position to know what type of professional help to seek, and to become a true partner in your health care when you find it. Starting points for that search are provided in the last chapter.

Okay, on with dealing with symptoms while you look for your particular causes!

2 SYMPTOM CONTROL
AS YOU DISCOVER CAUSE(S)

"Optimism is the faith that leads to achievement."

Helen Keller

L et's talk about symptom management during the time you're finding out what's causing your joints to become inflamed. In other words, buying yourself comfort while you discover a healing direction.

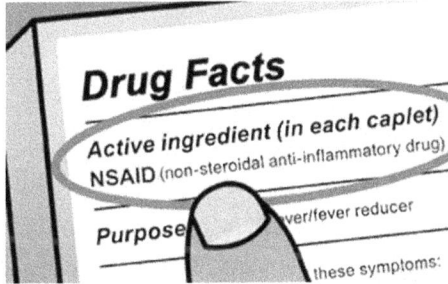

Drug Facts

Active ingredient (in each caplet)
NSAID (non-steroidal anti-inflammatory drug)

Purpose   ver/fever reducer

these symptoms:

**Figure 4 To find out if a drug is a NSAID, check the
Active ingredients label**

There are many over the counter pharmaceutical pain management products. Those for arthritis are generally in a category called "NSAIDS". Spelled out, this acronym means 'non-steroidal anti-inflammatories." The most commonly recognized drugs in this category are aspirin, ibuprofen and naproxen. In general these drugs reduce pain, decrease fever, and in higher doses, decrease inflammation. If your inflamed joint involves these enzymes, NSAIDS are likely to work for you to reduce your pain. Sounds great, right? Not so fast.

Before developing a habit of taking NSAIDS, inform yourself about their side effects, *especially from long-term use*. If they work for you, don't succumb to the temptation to think that if the pain is gone, the cause is also. Big mistake.

Especially concerning are three of the most common side effects: *heart attack, stroke and stomach bleeding*. Others include (but are not limited to) stomach pain, heartburn/ bleeding more easily/ headaches / dizziness / ringing in the ears/ liver, kidney and central nervous system problems. Also, NSAIDS *do not inhibit the progression of arthritis, and they do not prevent joint damage.* (2-1)

In short, NSAID's suppress inflammation at a cost: they block the transformation of cells broken down from injury or strain into the molecules that direct the resolution of the inflammation. The result: inflammation continues.

Another class of drugs is the glucocorticoids, which work by suppressing your immune system as well as working against inflammation. However, they also carry with them long term risks. (2-2)

If you are taking an arthritis drug, but don't know whether or not it's a glucocorticoid, check the label for any of the following:

- beclomethasone
- betamethasone
- budesonide
- cortisone
- dexamethasone
- hydrocortisone
- methylprednisolone
- prednisolone
- prednisone
- triamcinolone

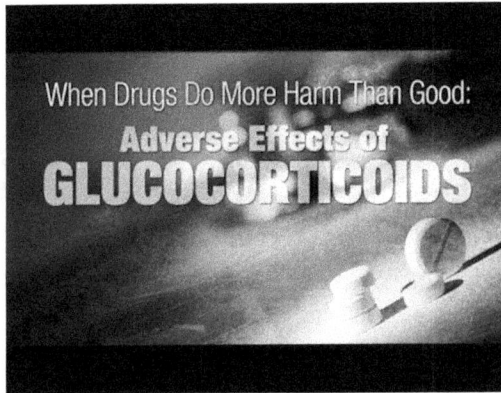

Figure 5 For more information on how these drugs can negatively affect you, check out this video: Negative Effects of Glucocorticoid Drugs

Does this mean then that you need either to endure pain or trade pain for such side effects? The short answer is, no. There are some key remedies–many that have been used in traditional cultures for hundreds of years–for such relief.

୨ଚ

WHAT YOU CAN DO

The Herbal Alternative

Boswellia. Boswellia is the primary herb used around the world for reducing arthritic inflammation. Native cultures have used Boswellia for centuries for this and other purposes. (2-3)

It is often used in combination with other herbs with anti-inflammatory properties, such as Turmeric, an herb in the ginger family that grows rhizomes instead of true roots. (2-4)

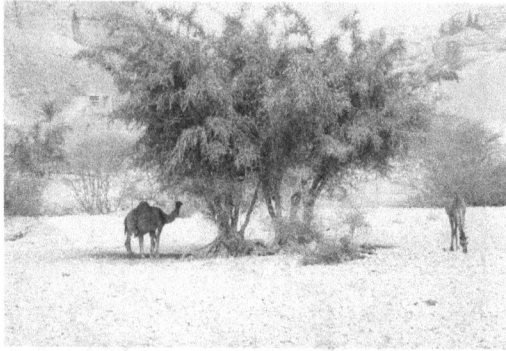

**Figure 6 This camel seems to know the benefits
of the Boswellia living tree, and not just for shade.**

Devil's Claw. This is another symptom-reducing herb that decreases pain and inflammation. (2-5)

Yucca Root. A third such herb is Mojave yucca root (Yucca schidigera,) also with anti-inflammatory properties.

White Willow Bark. Another herb specific for arthritic pain management is White Willow Bark. It's a natural source of salicin, flavonoids and other phenolic compounds that significantly reduce inflammation along with promoting joint health.

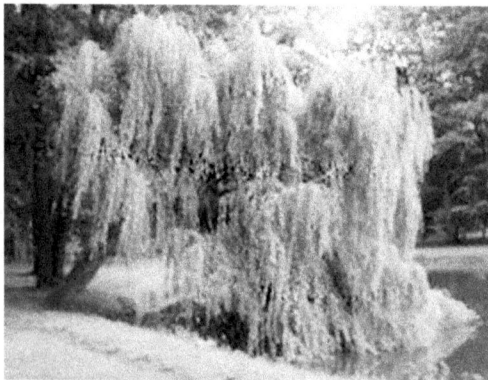

**Figure 7 This is a White Willow tree from which
white willow bark is harvested. This is the natural substance
from which aspirin is created in the laboratory.**

Proteolytic Enzymes. The above herbs may be combined with proteolytic enzymes that break down inflammatory molecules, such as Bromelain (from pineapple) or Papain (from papaya).

These enzymes are a top food element that can aid in the resolution of joint inflammation throughout your entire body, including your joints. Enzymes are catalysts that aid various biochemical processes in your body such as digestion, elimination and detoxification.

So significant are they that nutritional pioneer Royal Lee called arthritis a 'cooked food' disease. He noticed that arthritis-sufferers ate too much cooked food, and cooking destroys those enzymes. He encouraged people to eat more raw food, which contains those essential, inflammation-reducing enzymes in their active form.

Black Currant Seed Oil and Evening Primrose Oil. These oils are a component of foods called gamma linolenic acids, or GLA's. These oils act as natural anti-inflammatories because they provide the precursors your body needs to make its own anti-inflammatory molecules. They are found in the greatest concentration in black currant seed oil and in evening primrose oil.

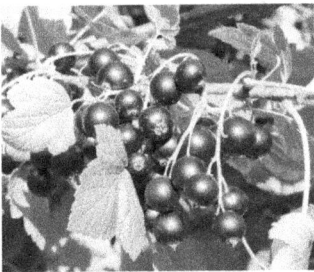

Figure 8 Black Currants on Vine

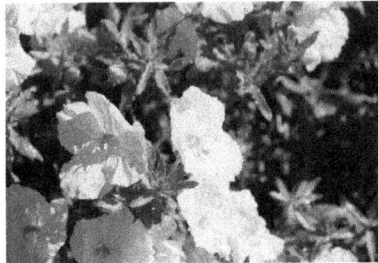

Figure 9 Evening Primrose Plant

These herbs, proteolytic enzymes and gamma linolenic acid can be used separately or in combination to relieve the *symptom* of joint inflammation.

In fact, doing so will put you in a much better frame of mind while you discover what might be causing your specific joints in your unique body to become inflamed.

So, before we can get into the specific causative factors in making those joints so painful, a reminder that the subjects below are not presented in any order (such as most likely to least likely, for example). Any one of them (or more than one) can be a at the root of your joint inflammation.

***

Endnotes:

2-1. These drugs work by inhibiting inflammatory enzymes, specifically COX-1 (cyclooxygenase-1) and COX-2 (cyclooxygenase-2).

2-2. Glucocorticoids "decrease calcium absorption and impair bone formation, leading to a significant decline in bone mineral density within the first 6–12 months of therapy. Additional side effects of sustained GC use include weight gain, redistribution of adipose tissue, and increased risk of developing diabetes mellitus, peptic ulcers, pancreatitis, cataracts, and glaucoma." Journal of Parasitology Research, Volume 2011 (2011), Article ID 942616, http://dx.doi.org/10.1155/2011/942616.

2-3. Now years of clinical research has revealed how Boswellia works: its boswellic acids reduce the formation of inflammatory leukotrienes.

2-4. Turmeric can stop inflammation by shutting down the COX2 enzymes that cause inflammation.

2-5. Devil's Claw said to be as effective as COX2 inhibiting drugs.

3. FOOD INTOLERANCES AND ALLERGIES

"The secret of getting ahead is getting started."
Sally Berger

Arthritis symptoms are very closely linked to the foods your particular body can handle, and also to the ones you've been requiring it to handle.

Which ones these are can vary both from person to person and from time to time; however there are some that you'll find are consistent across time. In part, that's because your unique DNA and blood type remain constant.

We'll talk about the most likely foods in a moment, but first, let's briefly cover a subject that can greatly affect inflammation throughout your body—especially those painful joints. It can also be confusing, so let's get it clarified now. It's about the difference between two terms: food intolerance and food allergy. They are significantly different from each other.

If you have a food intolerance, it means your body can't properly digest it. The symptoms caused by a specific food intolerance are the result of incomplete digestion (breaking down) of that food. This leaves undigested food particles floating around where they can cause inflammation, and one of those target organs is your joints.

A food allergy is different, however. A food allergen is a substance in a food that causes your immune system to put out danger signals and attack the substance. This is the cause of the symptoms it produces.

What's going on with an allergy is that your immune system is mistakenly identifying certain food ingredients – especially proteins- as if they were harmful invaders and then makes antibodies (immunoglobulin E, or IgE) against them. This is the start of a chain reaction, the downstream effect of which results in joint inflammation.

While food intolerances and food allergies are different, you can have them both concurrently. You might be intolerant of a food but not allergic to it, or allergic but not intolerant. Or you can be both intolerant of a food (unable to properly and completely digest it) _and_ allergic to it (meaning your body mounts an emergency alert reaction when you consume it).

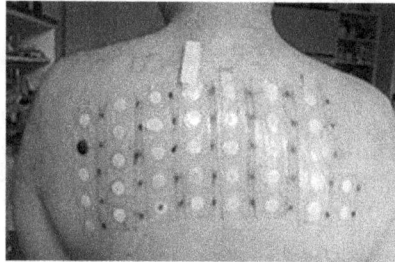

Figure 10 This man has had an allergy scratch test on his back. It will help determine his allergies but NOT his intolerances.

This is important to know because you might have a blood test or scratch test for a food _allergy_. This test is designed to reveal antigens. If your test shows no antigen for a particular food, it is assumed you're not allergic to it. However, _**you can still have a food intolerance**_.

Your intolerance will not be revealed by testing for antigens (because antigens are part of an _allergic_ reaction).
While continuing to ingest foods to which you are intolerant is definitely not good for your health, and particularly for your

arthritic symptoms, doing so is very unlikely to cause any *immediate* health danger. But ingesting food that causes an allergic reaction can create a medical emergency - a condition called anaphylactic shock. (3-1)

Now, unless there's an emergency, let's get on to some of the specific foods that can create arthritic inflammation.

$$\wp$$

WHAT YOU CAN DO

Reduce or Avoid *Saturated Fats* because they cause inflammation: Saturated fats may cause inflammation, especially if they are predominant over the unsaturated fats your body needs in approximately equal amounts. Saturated fats are found abundantly in meat (especially red meat) and dairy products.

Their balancers, the *un*saturated fats, are found in avocados, olive oil, safflower oil, peanuts, walnuts, a number of seeds, and fish such as salmon, trout, mackerel, tuna, sardines and herring.

Foods that are high in the saturated, or omega-6 fatty acids may increase inflammation, along with fatty and fried foods that contain trans-fats. These are present in dairy foods, which may also increase mucus production and gastrointestinal problems as well as contributing to inflammation in your body. (3-2)

Reduce or Avoid *High Glycemic Index* Foods because they cause inflammation: Sugar is at the top of the list of food elements that cause inflammation. That means that greatly reducing – even eliminating sugar – can have a positive effect on your inflamed joints.

Keeping your sugar intake low or even non-existent lowers your body's total inflammatory state, therefore reducing harmful effects all over your body, not just your joints.
Refined sugars and flours – especially white flour –are also top causes of joint inflammation. Sugar and other carbohydrates high in starch are called high-glycemic index foods. These definitely include high-sugar sodas, snack foods and baked goods. They can cause inflammatory problems because they fuel the production of advanced glycation end (AGE) products - and AGE's stimulate inflammation. (3-3)

Sugar cravings can be amazingly powerful, often winning even when you know better. One reason is that there are some infectious agents that have learned to make the neurotransmitters that can order your brain to eat carbos! Some of these infectious agents will be covered in chapters coming up. If you have sugar/ carbohydrate cravings, especially check out the section on Parasites and the one on Yeast, Fungus, Mold & Candida.

Reduce or Avoid *Wheat & Gluten* if they cause you inflammation: It seems like wheat is in everything these days, which is unfortunate because it's one of the primary foods that can cause joint inflammation. It doesn't matter how organically grown it is, how devoid of GMO's, how perfectly stone ground, how lovingly prepared, the bottom line is that it will cause inflammation if your body can't break it down. If you eliminate wheat from your diet, you may discover that not only do your arthritis symptoms disappear, but also that you drop weight quite naturally.

For other people, eliminating wheat is insufficient. What they need is to eliminate all sources of gluten. As you may recall, that's the sticky, gluey substance that holds bread together. If you suspect you may be gluten intolerant, you will need to eliminate all grains except these four: rice, amaranth, millet and quinoa. (We'll take up the subject of wheat again in Chapter 11.)

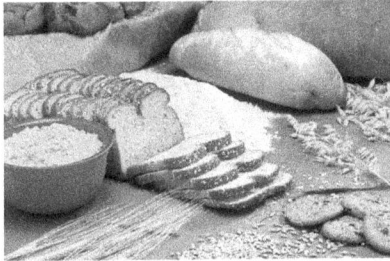

Figure 11 Even fresh, homemade bread with organic ingredients can cause major arthritic problems.

Reduce or Avoid *Nightshades* if they cause inflammation: This food group warrants particular attention because it can aggravate the pain and inflammation of arthritis. It includes tomatoes, white potatoes, eggplant, pepper, paprika and tobacco. Apparently the problem arises because they contain the chemical solanine. For some people, eliminating this food group has greatly reduced–and in some cases–even eliminated–joint pain and swelling. It's definitely worth your cutting it out from your diet as an experiment to see what effect it has for you. You may find you're not one of those affected. You just have to eliminate it for a around 3 weeks and find out what happens for you.

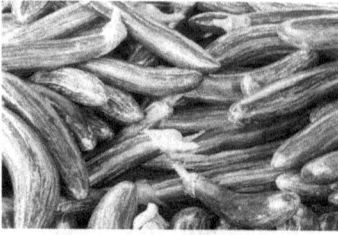

Figure 12 Japanese Eggplants, one of several varieties.

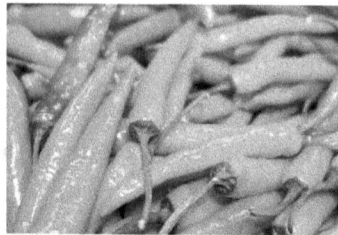

Figure 13 Pepper are all members of the nightshade family.

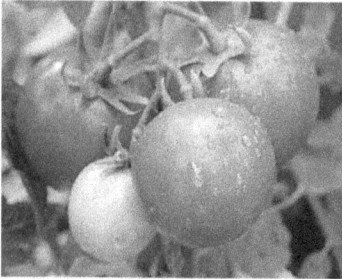

Figure 14 Tomatoes

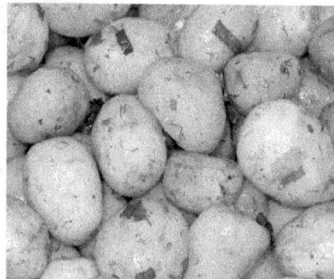

Figure 15 Potatoes

Some other substances in certain foods besides the ones mentioned above might be problematic for you, even if they're not an issue for the general population. Whether or not they are for you will depend to a large extent on your genetic inheritance. If you suspect some other foods are causing you joint inflammation, you can experiment by eliminating these other likely suspects: cow's milk, eggs, pork, codfish and strawberries. (3-4).

It's well worth pursuing the detective work it takes to discover any foods you need to eliminate from your diet. The bottom line is, once you get it right and stop consuming the foods that create inflammation for you, you will have made a major discovery that can put you on the road to restoring the health of your joints.

***

Endnotes:

3-1. If you suspect you or someone is having an allergic reaction that is leading to anaphylactic shock, you will need to act quickly, calling an ambulance to get you or them to the emergency room immediately. You (or they) might well require life-saving treatment. Since you don't know how severe the reaction will be, always err on the side of caution and notify the emergency team. Early signs include swelling that's developing rapidly, especially in the mouth or throat, trouble breathing, feeling dizzy, light-headed or faint. Don't guess – call 911.

3-2. http://www.livestrong.com/article/431059-nightshade-vegetables-and-arthritis-pain.

3-3. http://www.arthritis.org/living-with-arthritis/arthritis-diet/foods-to-avoid-limit/food-ingredients-and-inflammation-3.php.

3-4. https://www.docdoc.com/info/condition/allergic-arthritis.

4. Toxic Metals

"It always seems impossible until it's done."

Nelson Mandela

The situation with heavy metals in our world today is serious. Prior generations on this planet simply did not have this problem to the extent that we do. But even so there are ways of coming to grips with it and correcting it. Before we discuss the positive things you can do, let's spend a couple minutes understanding the essence of the problem.

No doubt you have some degree of heavy metal toxicity because that's almost impossible to avoid in this world. And no doubt you have some symptoms of metal toxicity, even though it's entirely likely you wouldn't recognize their cause. A toxic metal burden can cause an amazing number of symptoms that seem unrelated to each other. The questions for you, then, are "What is your toxic metal burden costing you?" And, "Is your toxic metal burden responsible for your arthritis?"

Toxic metals are those that poison your body and have no benefit for you. The four most common ones that are likely to affect you as a modern person are mercury, aluminum, lead and plutonium.

And, you're not exposed to just one metal. Your greatest toxic metal exposure comes from mercury, but you're also exposed to lead, aluminum, cadmium, even arsenic.

You might think you'd know when you're getting contaminated with toxic metals when it happens, but quite the reverse is true.

You don't know because the effects of toxic metals build up slowly over time, quite out of your awareness.

Possible sources of these contaminants are varied and depend on the metal itself. For example, two of the most common sources of mercury contamination are from dental amalgams, which are over 50% mercury, and vaccines containing Thimerisol, a preservative containing mercury. Other, less common toxic metals include antimony, uranium, arsenic, cadmium, barium, nickel and bismuth. Any of these can be deposited in the joints, stimulating inflammation.

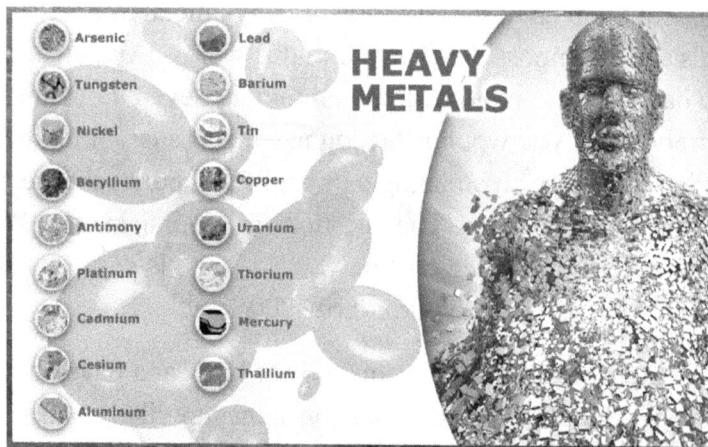

Figure 16 These are some toxic heavy metals that cause joint inflammation.

How Heavy Metals Cause Arthritis Heavy metals are the root cause of a number of diseases, not just arthritis. This chart below (created by Lyn Hanshew, M.D). illustrates them. (4-1) As you see, arthritis is right up there with the major illnesses. If you have any of the other diseases on this chart, and you also have arthritis, you should be doubly suspect that heavy metals are a major issue for you.

Inflammation is the cause of most major diseases

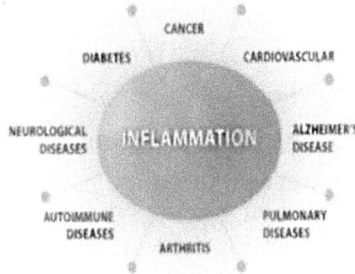

Correlation Between Toxicity and Inflammation!

The most effective course of action to reverse and prevent inflammatory symptoms is to DETOXIFY THE BODY from toxic heavy metals such as Mercury.
- Lyn Hanshew MD

Figure 17 Joint inflammation due to metal toxicity is a major contributor to arthritis

Here's one way arthritis from heavy metals can show their effect. If you're a young woman, your heavy metal burden can affect your family. That's because the single most effective force for removing those toxic metals from your body will be your unborn baby! Yes, to the extent that your body is contaminated, the little baby growing inside you will concentrate those toxic metals in its little body, and be born with a toxic metal burden before it even draws its first breath! (4-3)

And if its toxic metal burden is sufficient, the baby may be described as 'irritable'. It may be developmentally delayed, have trouble walking, talking, coordinating - in fact doing any kind of learning. And if you do what you're told is the 'right' thing, and you get all the recommended vaccinations for your child, you're having your child injected with more toxic metals from the vaccine!

Of course, pregnant women and their children are not the only ones that pay dearly for carrying a toxic metal burden. Many young children in school now are fighting to stay awake, fighting to retain their lessons, remember what they've learned, to build a second lesson on the first when they can't even remember what they had for breakfast, or whether they had breakfast.

They're told over and over to sit down, sit still, when their nervous systems are so short circuited from toxic metal exposure that all they can do, quite involuntarily, is jump around, flitting from one thing to the next without purpose or engagement in their world.

If their behavior is problematic enough for the school, they are labeled with a medical or psychiatric diagnosis and prescribed toxic medication on top of the toxic metal burden they're already carrying. (And if the child received Chinese medical herbs from China, they might also contain toxic metals).(4-4)

If you're an older person, you may fight against becoming more forgetful, or having more and more difficulty concentrating. You may even suffer gradual deterioration of your neurological functioning to the point where you're not safe to drive, until you can't even function independently anymore.

∿

WHAT YOU CAN DO

Replace Fear and Uncertainty with Reality. If any of these scenarios rings true for you, you might want to determine your toxic metal load. After all, you could spend a lot of time and energy that could be used to address whatever load you have with worry and fantasy about what your load might be.

A Self-Assessment. It's easy enough to start finding out the truth of your toxic metal load with a quick self-assessment. You can access a free toxic metals checklist at: www.freeoftoxicmetals.com.

Hair Analysis. You can also get a get a baseline hair analysis test, which many health care practitioners offer. They're also available online. Just search for" toxic metals hair analysis" . They are simple, but be sure to follow the directions accurately for preparing and collecting a snip of your hair to send to the lab for analysis.

Toxic Metals Challenge and Urine Sample. You can undertake a metals challenge. *__However, do this only under the direction of a health professional who is competent to advise you__*.

It involves taking a supplement—a chelating agent—that stimulates your body to release heavy metals. If they are present in your cells, the chelating agent will release them so they will appear in your urine. However, if you stimulate the release of heavy metals too quickly, you can become extremely ill. Again, carry this out only under the supervision of an experienced, competent health professional.

A urine sample following a metals challenge can look like this:

Toxic Metals; Urine

TOXIC METALS		RESULT µg/g creat	REFERENCE INTERVAL	WITHIN REFERENCE	OUTSIDE REFERENCE
Aluminum	(Al)	120	< 35		
Antimony	(Sb)	0.1	< 0.4		
Arsenic	(As)	49	< 117		
Barium	(Ba)	8.3	< 7		
Beryllium	(Be)	< dl	< 1		
Bismuth	(Bi)	0.6	< 15		
Cadmium	(Cd)	0.8	< 1		
Cesium	(Cs)	5.3	< 10		
Gadolinium	(Gd)	0.2	< 0.4		
Lead	(Pb)	7.3	< 2		
Mercury	(Hg)	21	< 4		
Nickel	(Ni)	12	< 12		
Palladium	(Pd)	< dl	< 0.3		
Platinum	(Pt)	< dl	< 1		
Tellurium	(Te)	< dl	< 0.8		
Thallium	(Tl)	0.4	< 0.5		
Thorium	(Th)	< dl	< 0.03		
Tin	(Sn)	0.4	< 10		
Tungsten	(W)	< dl	< 0.4		
Uranium	(U)	0.1	< 0.04		
URINE CREATININE		RESULT mg/dL	REFERENCE INTERVAL	-2SD -1SD MEAN	+1SD +2SD
Creatinine		84.3	35- 225		

Figure 18 Heavy metals challenge results

Limit Your Exposure. Even if you haven't done any assessments, you will still benefit by developing strategies for reducing your toxic metal burden by limiting your exposure.

To start, you can answer this question for yourself: "Where might I be exposed to these? " Then consider some of the places you're exposed to toxic metals. Here are some common sources of exposure followed by a couple suggestions for dealing with them:

• *The air you breathe:* Use a mask when working in a dusty environment; when in a car in traffic keep windows closed and run the fan; filter your air at home and clean/change the filter often.

• *The chemical 'fertilizers' used on the fields that grow your food;* eat organic food whenever possible; consider starting or expanding your own kitchen garden.

•*The amalgam fillings used to fill your teeth*: Make certain your dentist *never* uses any metal in repairing your teeth; get your amalgam fillings removed carefully by a mercury-free dentist. Check www.mercuryfree.com or www.dams.com 1.800.311.6265 or www.iaomt.org to locate one if needed.

• *The fish you eat from the streams and ocean:* Reduce your fish consumption, especially tuna fish. When you do consume it, choose from those species which are lower in mercury, such as: tilapia, shrimp, sardines, and Alaskan salmon.

• *The clothes you wear:* Choose clothes made of natural fabrics, such as cotton, hemp or linen. Make sure they're constructed free of toxic chemicals and dyes and heavy metals. One way is to make certain its Global Organic Textile Standard (GOTS) certified. You can also use their free database, a valuable resource, at GOTS free public database.(http://www.global-standard.org/public-database.html) In any case, wash all new clothing before wearing.

•*Paints, including those that outgas from your walls:* Choose paints with low 'volatile organic compounds', or low VOC paint. Use water-based products over solvent containing ones. Buy premixed paints. Avoid working with powered paints. Choose brushing and dipping techniques over spray methods. Plan studio ventilation with adequate air flow. Avoid dusty procedures. Avoid skin contact with paints by wearing gloves. Wear protective clothing and goggles if needed. Avoid eating, smoking, or drinking around work area. Dispose of waste paints and products in accordance with health and safety regulations. (4-2)

• *Some vaccinations you receive.* Supposedly mercury (as Thimerosol) was supposed to be removed from vaccines. However, some evidence exists that mercury is present even in single dose vaccines. Mercury content of currently used vaccines can be found at http://www.vaccinesafety.edu/thi-table.htm. If you can avoid getting a vaccine, do so. If you are required by law (or coerced by threats to your employment), work with health professional to detox yourself immediately after you receive it.

• *Exposure at work.* If you're concerned about exposure to a toxic metal, especially if you're employed where you fear toxic metal exposure, you may be interested in what the U.S. Government has to say about occupational exposure on the job. You can find exposure risks, exposure limits, and health effects at The Occupational Health and Safety website under 'heavy metals.' (4-3)

Heavy metals are such an important cause of joint inflammation that you may want to delve in to the subject more deeply. You can get a review of the essentials you need to know, including symptoms specific to women, to men, to children, neurological effects, immune effects, sources of specific heavy metal exposure, the variety of chelating agents and, most important, how to release your toxic metals burden *safely.*

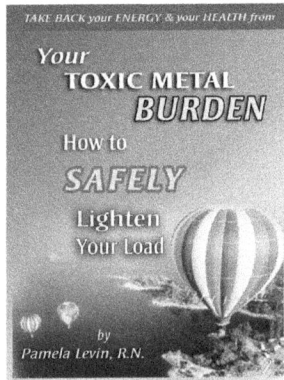

Figure 19 Releasing your toxic metal burden safely is crucial; otherwise you could become very ill. This book is one resource that tells you how.

***

Endnotes:

4-1. http://www.svhi.com/wp-content/uploads/2016/04/Lyn-Hanshew-MD-Oral-Heavy-Metals-Detox.pdf.

4-2. http://mercury.wm.edu/expo/wp-content/uploads/2008/10/heavymetals_and_paint.pdf

4-3. http://www.osha.gov/SLTC/metalsheavy/index.html.

4-3. https://www.nytimes.com/2017/06/01/opinion/toxic-chemicals-pregnancy-fetus.html.

4-4. http://www.businessinsider.com/study-reveals-chinese-medicines-contain-trace-amounts-of-toxic-substances-2015-12.

5. Synthetic Chemicals

"Life is 10% what happens to you and
90% how you react to it."
Charles Swindoll

As someone living in the 21st century, you are exposed to an ever- growing number of toxic chemicals. Luckily, there are some constructive and straightforward ways of dealing with this, but before we get to that, let's take a look at the reality, which, granted, is not very pretty. Still, it can motivate you to take some simple constructive steps that can make all the difference, so hang in there, and let's take a look.

Estimates – even conservative ones – calculate that if you're an average person, in your daily life you're exposed to well over 100,000 synthetic chemicals.

That's definitely bad news, but what makes it even more so is that the number is increasing: estimates are that you'll be exposed to about 1,000 more new chemicals that are added every year to the 85,000 already on the federal registry. (5-1)

One of the first groups of people to validate this was undertakers, who have for many decades now pointed out that the bodies of the deceased take much longer to decompose than they did prior to the use of preservatives in food. (5-2)

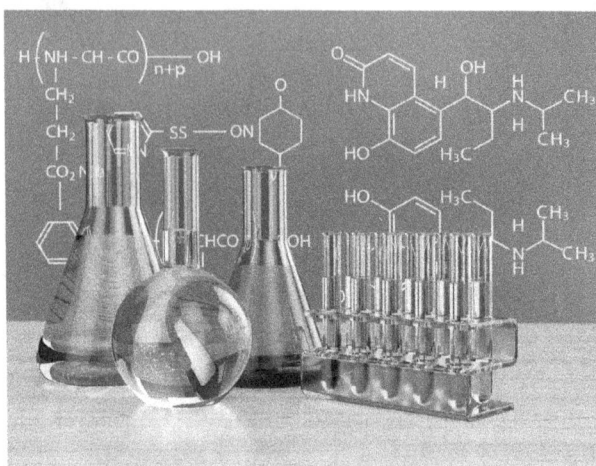

**Figure 20 Synthetic chemicals are those made
in the laboratory rather than by nature.**

The truth is, that for the first time in human history, you and everyone else, have become living, breathing, synthetic chemical experiments. Like others, your body now contains an enormous _mix_ of chemicals. In fact there's nowhere in the world where this can be avoided, due in part to jet stream, prevailing winds, countries and corporations dumping their chemical waste into the food supply, the soils, the air or the water.

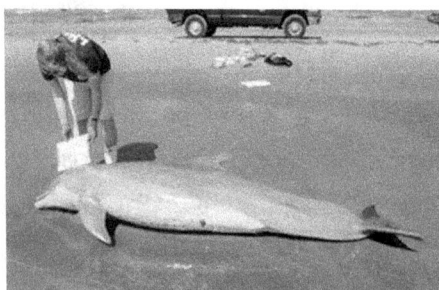

**Figure 21 Humans ultimately share the fate of this dolphin
because our bodies also carry a heavy load of synthetic chemicals.**

This massive exposure results in an immense body burden. In fact, it's way too significant for your liver to detoxify and eliminate on its own. Since these synthetic toxins can't be eliminated as rapidly as they are amassed, they back up in your body, and this can cause – you guessed it - joint inflammation.

How bad is it? The following graph depicts the rate of increase in your synthetic chemical exposure since 1955:

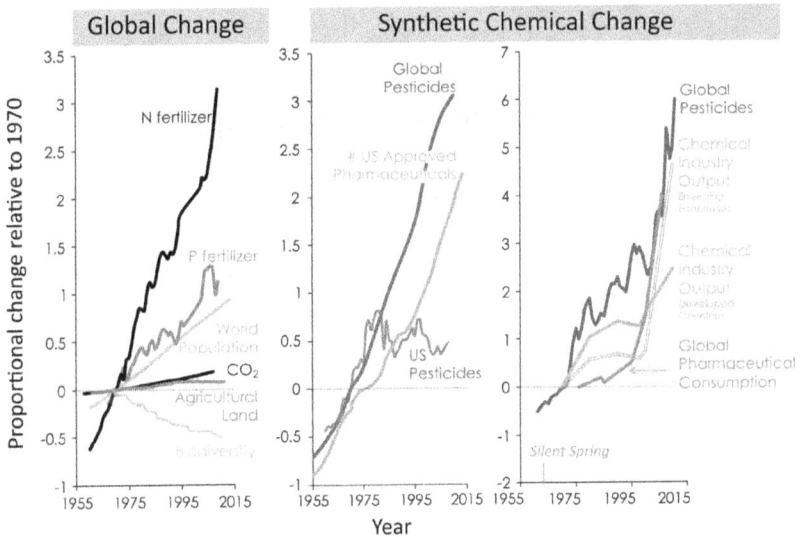

Figure 22 Rise in synthetic chemicals since 1955

Of the total number of synthetic chemicals, only a couple hundred have been tested for their effects on our health, and of those, fewer still have been checked for their effects of pregnant women, developing infants and children. This fact alone means that the health of each new generation may already be severely impacted.

Given that this is your condition, the worst thing you can do about it is to indulge yourself in 'the ostrich trick' - burying your head in the sand because you feel threatened. In this instance, out of sight is definitely not out of mind!

Luckily, you don't have to wait decades for the scientific community to prove - or the medical system to learn to diagnose – that the unique mix of chemicals in your body contributes to your physical problems. Nor do you need to wait while the governmental bodies dither over what regulations to impose – or even whether to impose them.

༉

WHAT YOU CAN DO

The following are ways to reduce your toxic chemical burden yourself. Each action is empowering, effective and constructive:

Your Home Environment:

The website *Popular Mechanics* recommends that you start in your home, especially. (5-4) They point out that the chemicals you're exposed to there are " 1,000 times as likely to be inhaled as outdoors." Here's how they suggest starting to reduce your home exposure:

Vent your gas stove outside to avoid releasing polycyclic hydrocarbons, created by incomplete combustion, into your home, says Shelly Miller, an air-pollution researcher at the University of Colorado.

Use minimal carpet and drapery. "Carpets can be a reservoir for all sorts of particles," Miller says.

Use a HEPA filter on your vacuum and heating system to keep captured particles from escaping back into the air.

Look up cosmetic and cleaning products on the Environmental Working Group's "Skin Deep" database (www.ewg.org), which rates more than 50,000 products on a scale of 0 (safe) to 10 (hazardous). You'll notice a reference to a "data gap" rating. This tells you whether the results are based on research carried out by the industry itself, or is actually independent comprehensive safety data.

Your Bodily Environment (5-5)

Eat organic foods whenever possible and avoid processed foods. These are major steps in cleaning up your bodily environment. They do your body a big favor by reducing the toxic load that enters it. Also, doing these two things is a political act because you're voting with your wallet. You're saying no to non-foods, fake foods and adulterated foods.

Technically speaking, the term 'organic' means grown without the use of pesticides, synthetic fertilizers, sewage sludge, genetically modified organisms, or ionizing radiation or animals that produce meat, poultry, eggs, and dairy products do not take antibiotics or growth hormones.(5-6)

However, if it's labeled "USDA Organic" it means 95% organic with the other 5% being who knows what.

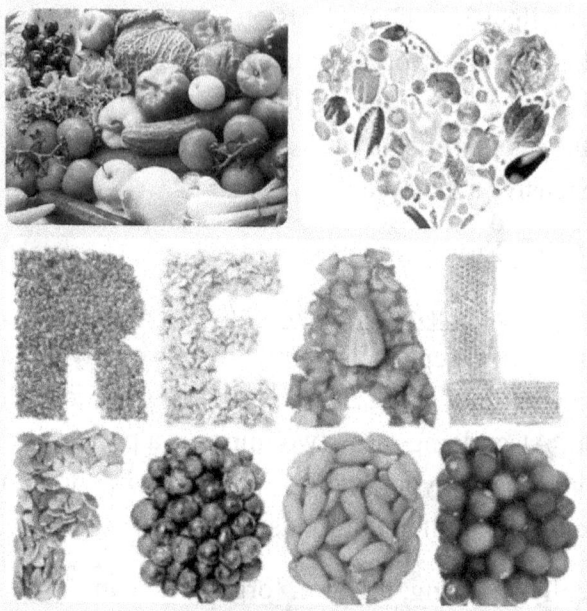

Figure 23 The names of real foods can make you salivate, while the names of synthetic foods do not.

Load Up on **Whole Food** B Vitamins Healthy DNA in every cell depends on whole food vitamin B. The best food source is Brewer's Yeast. But pay attention to the kind you buy: chemical companies are now buying up food companies and contaminating real food with fake vitamins. If you get a niacin rush (flushing, reddening of the skin, along with burning or itching), it means fake B's are present. Throw it out, and try a different source (probably one in a can rather than in the bulk food section).

Do NOT use synthetic vitamin B, as it can damage peripheral nerve plates and actually create heart arrhythmias and other nervous system disturbances.

Instead, read the label on the back of the Brewer's yeast jar. Under ingredients, it should list only Brewer's yeast, also called nutritional yeast. If it also lists any individual B vitamins, then they've added synthetic ones.

For example, looking at the ingredients of one brand, the front label used the word 'fortified' – a definite warning sign. The back, under ingredients, said the following: "Ingredients: Primary grown Nutritional Yeast (Saccharomyces cerevisiae), Niacin, Pyridoxine HCl, Riboflavin, Thiamine HCl, Folic Acid and Vitamin B-12." Every ingredient listed after Nutritional Yeast (Saccharomyces cervesisiae) is a synthetic B vitamin.

Bathe Your Cells in Generous Amounts of Anti-Oxidants Many chemicals damage DNA. To defend your DNA from this damage, employ antioxidants. Especially important are vitamins A, C and E, but again, use only whole food sources. Carrots and fresh carrot juice are a rich source of natural, whole food vitamin A.

A great source of whole food vitamin C is the juice of a lemon squeezed into filtered water. But don't buy or use ascorbic acid. It's what government standards call vitamin C, but that's only one part of the whole vitamin C complex nature made. Instead, it is a laboratory concoction made by boiling sulfuric acid and corn syrup together. Ascorbic acid is actually the 'wrapper' that protects the payload of vitamin C inside – it's equivalent to eating the banana peel and throwing away the banana.

Whole food vitamin E, which is free of the negative effects being discovered by the synthetic isolates of vitamin E, is found in wheat germ oil as well as fresh nuts and seeds. The amount to consume depends on your body's needs at the time. Organic wheat germ oil is sometimes used for therapeutic purposes. These doses are best determined by your health professional

Do not take synthetic isolates of vitamin E - they are toxic to your liver, and if only some are present, the ones you ingest will rob your body of the other parts to make it 'whole', thus creating deficits of the other parts.

Keep Yourself "Well-Oiled" Since chemicals and radiation deplete your body of essential fatty acids (EFA's, or vitamin F) you'll need to actively resupply them. In the space of about a month, you need roughly equal amounts of omega 3's., omega 6's and omega 9's. Most food sources contain a mix of these oils, which can be found in flax, chia, walnut, pumpkin and hemp seeds, dairy fats and legumes. We'll cover this topic in more detail in Chapter 13.)

An added benefit of providing plenty of these balanced fats is that they help you attain and maintain a normal weight. Avoid low fat diets; every cell and function of your body requires fats to function and stay healthy, starting with your brain, which is made of some 80% fat.

Keep Your Elimination Pathways Open Drink copious amounts of pure water to keep your system flushed. If you're not used to it, take the time to train yourself. Eight large glasses a day is excellent.

Exercise. Among its numerous benefits is the fact that it makes you sweat, and that flushes your system. Make it a point to sweat regularly and thoroughly. If you can't exercise for some reason, sit in a sauna.

Consume plenty of organic fiber. Fiber acts like a broom to sweep away toxins as they're released into your colon. Fruits,

38

vegetables and grains are an excellent source of fiber. Some experts recommend 70 grams of fiber a day for the average adult. That seems like a lot to most people.

There are also numerous fiber products on the market. Psyllium seed is one; however, if you're one of the many people who find it to be too harsh, check out the more gentle fibers such as those made from apple or grapefruit pectin.

Consume probiotic foods and/ or supplements. Adding probiotics (healthy bugs) is another way to support chemical detoxification. That's because probiotics help make sure your colon has the right bacteria to help digest what comes through. A great deal is being discovered now about which bacteria are the most beneficial and for what condition. Meanwhile a label on a typical probiotics supplement mind include such Lactobacillus strains as acidophilus, L. paracasei, L. caseei, and strains of Bifidobacterium.

You can also get these from cultured yoghurt, provided the product still contains live culture. Unfortunately there's no way to tell this from looking at the product or the label.
One strategy is to buy only kosher yoghurt, as the way most brands are processed keeps the live culture.

Fermented foods are another excellent source: sauerkraut, Natto, kefir, kombucha, tempeh, kimchi, pickles and lassi.

Provide Plenty of Sulfur Sulfur is essential for detoxification. Here's why: Your liver has two metabolic pathways it uses to detoxify anything your body needs to eliminate, and both those pathways use sulfur.

A good food source of sulfur is garlic. It protects against damage from free radicals that damage body tissues, helps maintain normal cholesterol and triglyceride levels and a healthy flow of blood through the circulatory system.

Other food sources include vegetables such as broccoli, cauliflower, cabbage, Brussel sprouts, watercress, kale, collard greens and radishes.

Consider Using Herbs That Support Detoxification A great variety of herbs exist that support detoxification in various ways. In choosing an herb, first make certain that it is organic. Many herbs (such as some imported from China) have been found to be contaminated with metals, and many from the US have been sprayed with pesticides.

If you use these, you will be spending your money to add an additional source of contamination.

Then, choose the right herb for the job. For that, you may require the services of a holistic health professional who has access to whole organic, therapeutic strength herbs and knows how to evaluate whether you need to detox from pesticides, food additives or what. (See the last chapter for ways to find such a professional.)

Some herbs, Chlorella, for example, can help detoxify your body of environmental pollutants from food, air and water because its cell wall attracts and binds with hydrocarbon pesticides and insecticides such as DDT, PCB and Kepone. This enables your body to carry them out -to eliminate them. Be forewarned however, Chlorella is a very powerful detoxifier and can cause a toxic release flood, so check with your holistic health professional before taking a Chlorella product.

If you need to detoxify your colon, then organic Spanish Black Radish is a good detoxifier to choose. It's also good for reducing liver congestion, diarrhea, viral load and constipation. It's high in sulfluothane, which grabs cancer cells.

Clues you might need to detoxify your colon is gum disease, unexplained weight gain, fatigue, muscle weakness and sleep disturbances.

Still other herbs are immune system boosters, blood cleansers, liver function supporters, bile production enhancers, promoters of cellular health, and so on. They have names like Echinacea, Turmeric, Andrographus, Ginger and Dandelion Root.

Homeopathic Remedies These are far ranging in their ability to help the body release toxins. Many are formulated specific to the toxin. One word of caution: many homeopathics are prepared in a base of lactose, so if you're lactose intolerant, be sure to check before taking any. In the United States, no homeopathic remedy can be marketed unless it is carried on a base of lactose. For this reason you may want to use liquid homeopathics, which don't have this problem.(5-7)

Know When to Get Competent Help If you're having symptoms of toxicity, it may be time to seek the services of a competent health professional. You can get yourself into a lot of trouble by trying to detoxify yourself by yourself.

Cloudy thinking, inability to make good choices, lassitude, lack of motivation and inability to follow through are all symptoms of toxicity. When you're already in that state and then stimulate your body to release even more toxins, you can become profoundly ill, especially when releasing very damaging substances such as heavy metals and certain chemicals.

A competent professional can assess your particular state of toxicity, monitor how quickly or slowly you need to detoxify and from what, choose the right products, whether herbs, homeopathics or whole food concentrates, determine your food intolerances and help you avoid further toxicity.

(Note: Again, check the last chapter for ways to find the health professional you need.)

With the current state of research and grant money, it would be very difficult to connect a specific chemical with a specific symptom such as arthritis. Nonetheless, by systematically detoxifying, you'll definitely think better, function better, have more energy and feel better. You'll bring your body pH into a more joint-friendly state. And, you will lower your risk of a variety of health problems, including not just arthritis, but even cancer. And that's worth a lot.

***

Endnotes:

5-1. http://popsci.com/science/article/2009-10/personal-chemistry#page-2.

5-2. Personal communication.

5-3. http://www.greenpeace.nl/Global/nederland/report/2007/6/human-impacts-of-man-made-chem.pdf.

5-4. https://www.popularmechanics.com/science/environment/news/a18841/toxic-chemical-discovered-in-san-Francisco's-fog/

5-5. This section excerpted from *Your Chemical Body Burden - What You Don't Know Can Hurt You*, http://www.betterhealtbytes.com/Volume-2-Issue-16.html.

5-6. Definition from www.organic.org.

5-7. Homeopathic remedies exist for cellular release of tobacco, dust, hydrocarbons, molds, radiation (such as U.V., microwaves, radon, cobalt, x-rays, TV's video display terminals and geopathic disturbances), sulfur dioxide, sulphurous acid (the principle ingredient in acid rain), heavy metals, residual toxins from infections (bacterial, viral, yeast, parasite, or nematode), food additives (food colorings, flavorings, preservatives, sweeteners, acidulents, bleaches, emulsifiers, humectants and thickeners, hormones, leavenings and solvents such as acetone and hexane), insecticides, phenolics and dental materials (alloys containing chromium, copper, nickel, silver, tin, zinc, mercury, cements, resents, chlorine and fluoride.

6. LYME & LYME VECTORS
"Every accomplishment starts with the decision to try.

No doubt you've heard horror stories – or even had the displeasure of experiencing it yourself – people spending sometimes even years on antibiotics and still not getting free of Lyme disease.

So please be reassured that there are things you can do to help prevent it, and to address it effectively if you need to – and without antibiotics. Let's take a moment to find out what it actually is, and then we'll get to the constructive steps you can take.

How can a bite from a tiny insect tick - no larger than the period at the end of this sentence – cause such profound health challenges?

Yet that is exactly what happens when you receive a tick bite so subtle you're likely not even to notice it. But the tick injects infectious agents into your body through its saliva. As a group, these infectious agents are all referred to as 'Lyme vectors'. And the most dreaded term – Lyme disease.

As it's usually used the term 'Lyme disease' may refer to only one of a number of arthritis-causing infections carried by tick bites – the one caused by a spiral-shaped bacteria (hence the name 'spirochete'). This kind is from the bacteria Borrelia burgdorferi, or Bb), and it causes a form of infectious arthritis.

Anyone can get Lyme disease but it is more common in children. In fact, when this form of Lyme disease began to spread on the East Coast of the United States, doctors from Yale University who were assigned to investigate, misdiagnosed thirty-nine children as having juvenile arthritis, failing to recognize that they were seeing a form of infectious arthritis.

The Borrelia spirochete bacteria is carried by a small tick (called Ixodes or deer tick) that lives on deer and mice. It is found in wooded areas during the spring and early summer. Many areas of the US have reported cases of Lyme disease. However most cases occur in seven states: New York, New Jersey, Rhode Island, Connecticut, Massachusetts, Wisconsin and Minnesota. (6-1)

Ticks feed on mice and other animals all through the year, and as these animals move into new habitats, the ticks, with their Lyme disease, move with them. So rapidly is this form of Lyme disease proliferating, that maps have been made for veterinarians to predict its spread. Because dogs are also infected, the hope is that this information can be used to help track and predict it in people. The following is the prediction for dogs in 2017: (6-2)

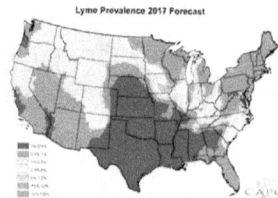

Lyme Prevalence 2017 Forecast

Figure 24 Map predicting 2017 spread of Lyme disease in the U.S.

☙

WHAT YOU CAN DO

To protect yourself from Lyme disease when you visit wooded or lake areas, use the suggestions below. as these measures may help prevent tick bites (6-3)

- wear long sleeves and pants;
- pull socks over pant legs;
- wear closed shoes;
- wear a hat;
- use tick repellent on clothes;
- shower afterwards and inspect for ticks particularly checking arms, legs and hairline.

If you are bitten by a tick, you may not see it at all initially because it is very tiny, no larger than a pinhead or match head. It is oval and has eight legs.

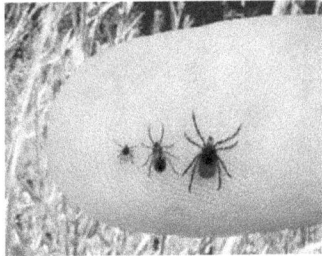

Figure 25 Size of tick nymph, adult female and male, respectively, on a human finger.

When the tick bites you, it injects the spirochete into your blood stream and begins to feed. This phase is when you may start to notice it, for its blood meal can cause it to swell to 100 times its initial size.

Remove it carefully. This is the time to remove it _properly._ If you try to remove it with your hands, it will expose you to the infectious load the tick might be carrying. Instead, use tweezers, and then carefully disinfect the tweezers after removing the tick.

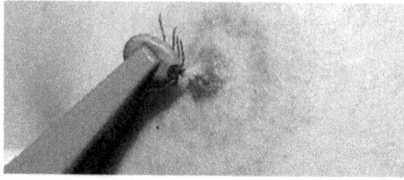

Figure 26 How to remove a Lyme tick.

Check for the rash. If you don't experience any immediate symptoms, don't relax yet. Symptoms of Lyme Bb infection usually don't appear until 1-3 weeks after you're bitten. This is when you may start to feel those aching, arthritic joints, and may start to see the classic bull's-eye Lyme rash, which looks like this:

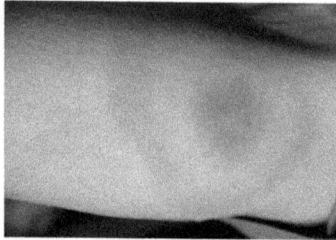

**Figure 27 Classic Lyme rash following bite from infected tick.
Remember, not all Lyme infections begin with this rash.**

However, if this classic rash doesn't appear, it still does _not_ necessarily mean that you're not infected. In other words, you may still be infected.

Check for early symptoms. Check for these other symptoms of early Lyme disease: (6-4)

The aforementioned skin rash, 5-20 inches in diameter, with a white center that's hard and hot, surrounded by redness, white in the center and bright red on the outside. It's usually around the bite, but can appear on various areas of your body, and can last up to a month.

- Flu-like symptoms of fever and chills, fatigue, headache, vomiting and soreness all over.
- Joint pain and swelling usually in your knees and sometimes also hips, shoulders and ankles.
- Sore throat, dry cough, stiff neck, swollen glands.
- Dizziness and sensitivity to sunlight.

Seek help from your health professional right away. If you have these symptoms, don't delay. With immediate treatment and the correct medication, this form of Lyme disease can be resolved in a fairly short time. However, without this, symptoms can become more severe and recur several times over a year or more. That's because the Lyme spirochete takes on different forms and phases like another of its relatives in the spirochete family–syphilis.

If you are infected, but did not receive treatment, it's possible that the spirochete may ultimately spread to your brain, heart and nervous system over time. This is the stage of _chronic arthritis_ and may also include symptoms such as:

- temporary paralysis of your face;
- numbness and tingling in your hands or feet;
- severe headaches, depression, memory lapses;
- migrating pains in joints and tendons that come and go;
- stiff, aching neck;
- vertigo, dizziness;
- sleep disturbances;
- mental fogginess;
- problems following conversations and processing information;
- poor muscle coordination and
- heart problems.

Get the proper tests. To avoid this and receive a correct diagnosis, the Global Lyme Alliance recommends that you ask your doctor to order two tests: the blot test and the ELISA test. If they are positive, and if you've sought the help of an MD, you'll likely be offered a round of antibiotics, possibly even a number of kinds of antibiotics. with the aim of finding the right one.

Take probiotics if taking antibiotics. If you take antibiotics, remember that they will kill off a whole range of healthy bugs in your G.I. tract (your Microbiome) and you will need to replace these with probiotics supplements taken long-term in order to protect your health.

Effective herbs and herbal combinations. If your health practitioner is a naturopath, acupuncturist, chiropractor, herbalist etc. you may be offered some particular herbs or herbal combinations that can assist your body in clearing the infection.

For example, herbalists in Australia, who also have to contend with Lyme, might use the herb Sweet Wormwood, which contains Artemisinin. It was discovered when malaria suffers' symptoms were reversed in only 6 days.(6-5). Many also combine it with Sarsaparilla root, Stemona root, Black Walnut Hull extract and/or Clove bud.

If you find you've improved some with treatment, but you still have some symptoms, the tick bite may have injected you with other infective agents which are part of the variety of Lyme vectors. Happily, the above herbs and herbal combinations also prove effective against them.

Herbs and mushrooms for viral Lyme vectors. The exception is if you have a viral infection caused by a tick bite. There are no effective pharmaceutical products for viral problems; however there are many herbs and herbal combinations that can support your body in eliminating them.

As viruses don't respond to antibiotics, you will find the best remedies among herbs and mushrooms. Among those that support the body in eliminating viruses include St. John's Wort (especially effective against envelope viruses), Andrographus, Cat's Claw, Burdock Root, Sheep Sorrel and Sarsaparilla. Some viruses are eliminated with the support of mushrooms such as Ganoderma and Shitake. Also check Chapter 8, where we address viral causes of arthritis more specifically.

Whatever the Lyme vector or remedy, you'll no doubt agree that the best bet is to avoid tick bites altogether. And hopefully you're reassured, that whatever infective agent might be injected into you when you are bitten, there are effective remedies at hand.

***

Endnotes:

6-.1 https://www.cdc.gov/lyme/stats/index.html.

6-2. Ibid.

6-3. https://www.mayoclinic.org/diseases-conditions/lyme-disease/symptoms-causes/syc-20374651

6-4. https://www.cdc.gov/lyme/signs_symptoms/index.html

6-5. https://www.ncbi.nlm.nih.gov/pmc/articles/PMC2901398.

7. PARASITES

"Problems are not stop signs, they are guidelines."
Robert Schuller

It's likely all you had to do was read the title of this section and you had the typical reaction: "Eww!" Not surprising if you did, because most people association having a parasite problem with being unclean. Unfortunately, being clean is insufficient protection against these invaders.

Also you might think that being a citizen of a Western country would protect you. Here's a pop quiz: if you had to guess what world country has the biggest parasite problem, what would you answer? A likely guess would be Africa, right? Well, that would be wrong!

According to Dr. Frank Nova, Chief of the Laboratory for Parasitic Diseases of the U.S. National Institute of Health, "In terms of numbers, *there are more parasitic infections acquired in this country [the United States] than in Africa*". (7-1)

The chief of Patho-Biology at Walter Reed Army Institute of Research, Dr. Peter Wina, concurs. "We have a tremendous parasite problem right here in the U.S., it is just not being addressed," he says. (7-2.) As strange as that might be to believe, still, you might wonder, what does that have to do with the subject at hand? In other words, how do parasites relate to arthritis? In short, plenty.

So hang in there, and let yourself get past that "Eww!" response. Because parasites have everything to do with arthritis. Once you realize the facts, hopefully you'll hang in there to access the following section about what you can do. Here are some ways:

- Parasites can migrate to your joint fluids where they encyst (become enclosed in a sac) in joint fluids (they can also encyst in muscles). Once this happens, the resulting pain becomes manifest and is diagnosed as arthritis. They may exist in some joints but not others.
- Parasite waste products and the toxins they produce can gather in your joints, creating inflammation and pain.
- Parasites can cause tissue damage in your joints, to the point of actually eroding them in some cases.
- Joint and muscle pains and inflammation can also result from your body's ongoing immune response to their presence. (7-3)
- The above are effects of direct infection of a joint. Indirectly, parasites can set up symptoms of gouty arthritis by impairing your kidney function, resulting in increased uric acid which accumulates in joints, forms crystals and cause flare-ups of gout. (See Chapter 14.)
- Parasites can cause your body to become confused, thus attacking your own joints. This form of arthritis is called autoimmune arthritis (see Chapter 16.)
-

Since parasites can cause arthritis, you might wonder, "Why doesn't my immune system mount an effective immune response and kill off the little buggers?"

Scientists have also wondered about this. After studying this very question, they conclude that, "Worm parasites have co-evolved with the mammalian immune system for many millions of years and during this time, they have developed extremely effective strategies to modulate and evade host defenses and so maintain their evolutionary fitness." (7-4)

$$\wp$$

WHAT YOU CAN DO

At last, we can discuss effective way to eliminate parasites. That said, the effective ways depend both on the parasite itself, including the stage (or form) of its evolution (egg, larvae, adult) and its location in its unwilling host. All these factors together are what makes it so difficult to deal with them effectively. That said, there are a number of ways to go about it, and for any one parasite, a number of them may be required.

First, there are a number of pharmaceuticals available by prescription. This approach requires a medical diagnosis. That can be difficult to obtain for two reasons. One, because typical diagnosis relies on laboratory tests of stool samples, and two, if the critter doesn't happen to locate itself in your gut at the moment your body produces the sample the test will come back negative when you really do have a problem.

Meanwhile, its progeny are happily hijacking your food before you even have a chance to get at it, making your brain crave things you know aren't good for you (lots of carbohydrates, for example) and possibly even munching away at your joints, causing your arthritic symptoms.

Too, pharmaceuticals have side effects, and these can be daunting in some cases. For example, the recommended drug for one such critter relies on inhibition of folic acid. Blocking folic acid results in the critter not being able to continue making more DNA, thus rendering it incapable of reproducing itself.

This sounds great, however, the problem is that it also prevents YOU from being able to replicate your own DNA, and that means you can't make new cells to replace old and dying ones.

There are also many non-pharmaceutical approaches which are largely from the realm of herbs, concentrated nutritional supplements and mushrooms. None of these has side effects, but only effects.

Some that have been demonstrated to be clinically effective include the following, used either alone or in combination with others mentioned:

- Sarsaparilla
- Burdock Root
- Wormwood (and its constituent Artemesian)
- Black Walnut Hulls
- Protein-digesting enzymes on an empty stomach
- Wheat Germ Oil (most effective on empty stomach)
- Certain concentrated mineral products.

To sort through all this by yourself would be daunting indeed, which is why it's best to find a competent practitioner who can not only assess your particular health needs, but also has ways to discover parasite issues (muscle testing, for example), find the particular remedies your body needs and know when these need to change. For example, one remedy may be required for eliminating the adult form in your gut, but another entirely for the eggs in your joints. (See Chapter 18 on Finding Professional Help.)

OK, good for you! You've gotten this far. Hopefully you can tolerate just a bit more managing your "Eww!" response, because the next section will acquaint you with three of the most significant invaders. The first two are the most likely suspects when it comes to the connection between infectious arthritis and parasites, while the third applies especially to rheumatoid arthritis.

Once you gain this brief understanding of them, you'll be in a much better position to watch out for them, and to gain the upper hand if necessary. And that can only bode well for resolving your arthritis.

Here's the first one:

Infectious Arthritis and Strongyloides stercoralis. The fact that arthritis symptoms can be caused by this parasite was amply demonstrated by the medical faculty of a university hospital in Adana, Turkey who authored a case report. In aspirating fluid from an arthritis joint, they literally found a particular parasite in the fluid: Strongyloides stercoralis. (7-5)

Direct infection of joints was also proven when the synovial fluid in an ankle joint was aspirated with a needle. Again, the fluid disclosed Strongyloides infection. (7-6)

Here's what Strongyloides stercoralis looks like:

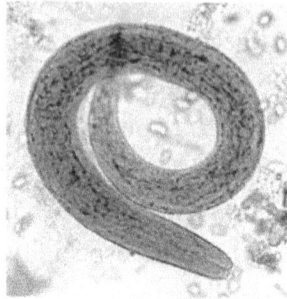

Figure 28 This little worm can wreak havoc in your joints.

This is the most researched of the various parasites and the one most strongly implicated in directly causing joint inflammation."Strongyloides stercoralis is a human pathogenic parasitic roundworm causing the disease strongyloidiasis. Its common name is threadworm."

According to the CDC "*Strongyloides* is known to exist on all continents except for Antarctica, but it is most common in the tropics, subtropics, and in warm temperate regions. The global prevalence of *Strongyloides* is unknown, but experts estimate that there are *between 30–100 million infected persons worldwide*." (7-7)

According to the U.S. Centers for Disease Control (CDC), "The global prevalence of Strongyloides is unknown, but experts estimate that there are *between 30–100 million infected persons worldwide*." (7-8)

According to the scientists who research it, "The persistence of infection, increasing international travel, lack of familiarity by health care providers, and potential for hyper infection all make Strongyloidiasis an emerging infection to reckon with." (7-9)

This clever little invader has a life pathway that helps it not only survive, but thrive in humans. Here's how it works:

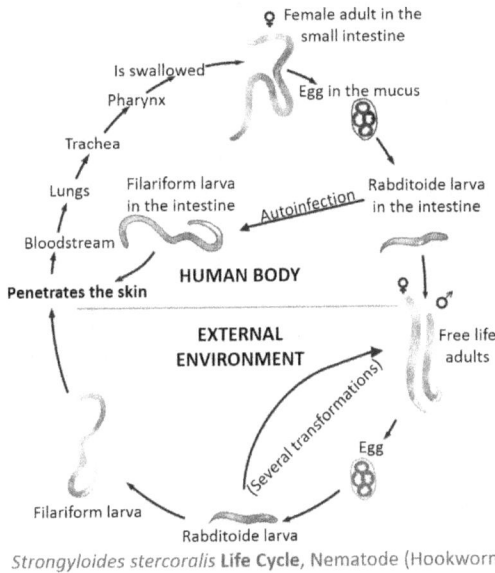

Female adult in the
small intestine

Is swallowed

Pharynx

Trachea

Lungs

Filariform larva
in the intestine

Bloodstream

Penetrates the skin

Egg in the mucus

Rabditoide larva
in the intestine

Autoinfection

HUMAN BODY

**EXTERNAL
ENVIRONMENT**

Free life
adults

Several transformations

Egg

Filariform larva

Rabditoide larva

Strongyloides stercoralis **Life Cycle**, Nematode (Hookworm)

**Figure 29 This parasitic hookworm, Strongyloides stercoralis, has
several stages that help it hide and survive in humans.**

To avoid infection, or reinfection, consider the following
precautions:

- Don't walk with bare feet;
- Avoid contact with human waste or sewage, and if
  you are, wear protective gloves, then engage in
  vigorous hand washing after;
- If your occupation increases contact with
  contaminated soil such as farming and coal mining,
  wear protective clothing, including masks so soil
  dust can't enter your lungs;
- If you travel internationally, consider taking a
  preventative protocol during travel and after.

Infectious Arthritis and Trichuris trichuria. Let's take a
closer look at one of the most common and highly infectious

parasites. Its Latin name is Trichuris trichuria. Its common name is whipworm. If you are infected with it, you probably got an egg from soil that was contaminated when feces were used in a fertilizer, for example, or when a person or animal already infected defecates outside.

Here's what they look in their egg form:

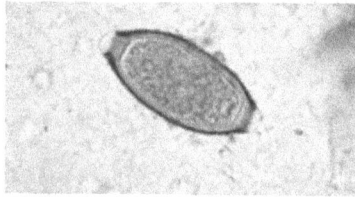

Figure 30 The highly infectious Trichuris trichuria in egg form.

When the eggs hatch and mature into adults, they look like this:

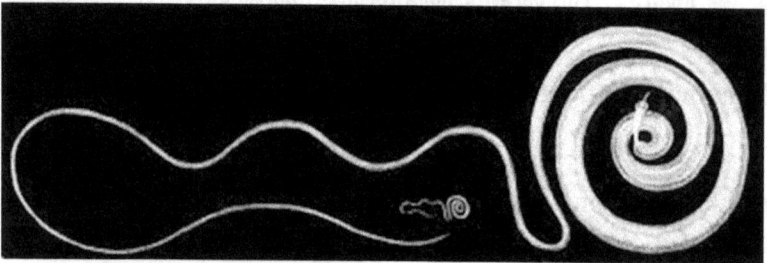

Figure 31 Trichuris trichuria in the adult whipworm stage.

This female whipworm, once in your intestines, can produce 2,000–10,000 single-celled *eggs per day.* Imagine those now travelling to the soft tissue in your body, landing in your joints and deciding to take up residence.

Again according to the CDC (U.S. Centers for Disease Control) the best way to prevent whipworm infection and also the above-mentioned hookworm, is to always:

Avoid ingesting soil that may be contaminated with human feces, including where human fecal matter ("night soil") or wastewater is used to fertilize crops.

Wash your hands with soap and warm water before handling food.

Teach children (and remind adults about) the importance of washing hands to prevent infection.

Wash, peel, or cook all raw vegetables and fruits before eating, particularly those that have been grown in soil that has been fertilized with manure.

Roundworms and Rheumatoid Arthritis. This painful condition has long been known to result from a bacterial infection. What's news is that scientists have discovered that the bacteria that inflame the joints actually come from larger parasites. In other words, the parasites – little wormlets actually living in the joints - are themselves infected with bacteria.

This kind of parasite is a common type of little roundworm whose eggs hatch into microscopic wormlets that travel. The most frequently found such invaders that can cause arthritis in this way are four common roundworms: Ascaris, Hookworm, Strongyloides and Trichinella. (7-10)

The point is, that once you've cleared the parasite infection, either with pharmaceuticals or with the herbs etc. mentioned above (or both!), you may also need to get on a protocol for a bacterial infection.

That may sound like a lot of work, and daunting, but when you consider the possibility of becoming free from arthritis as a result, perhaps you will feel more motivated to hang in there and get this resolved.

Plus, keep in mind that these little invaders don't limit themselves to causing arthritis only; they can cause a variety of other health difficulties, so any effort you make to rid yourself of them can only work in favor of your long term health and well-being.

Lastly, you should know that even though parasites are definitely implicated in arthritis, a recent focus of research has been on using them to _treat_ arthritis:

"The consideration of the impact of infection with helminth parasites on arthritic disease is limited, but the available data support the general concept of _"helminth therapy"—or rather, that data obtained from models of arthritis and concomitant helminth infection have the potential to reveal novel approaches to treat arthritis."_ (7-11)

If this sounds like a doubtful approach to you, remember that you must give _informed_ consent, and to truly be informed you should do your own research. Doctors are people too, and they can be like kids with a new toy when a new treatment approach becomes available. If you rely on them to inform you, you may not recognize the difference between child-like enthusiasm couched in medical terminology, and actual science-based facts that include all the downsides as well.

***

Endnotes:

7-1. https://www.yeastinfectionadvisor.com/humanparasites.html.

7-2. http://www.angelaburleson.com/parasites.html.

7-3. Ibid.

7-4. Parasitic worms. P Zaccone,* Z Fehervari,* J M Phillips, D W Dunne, and A Cooke.

7-5. Annals of the Rheumatic Diseases, 1984, 43, 523-525 Case report Parasitic arthritis induced by Strongyloides stercoralis . Akoolu, I. Tuncer, E., Erken, A,. Guray, F., L. Ozer, and K. Ozcan From the Department of Internal Medicine and Department of Pathology, f7ukurova University, Medical Faculty, Adana, Turkey.

7-6. Annals of the Rheumatic Diseases, 1984, 43, 523-525. http://ard.bmj.com/ on October 4, 2017 - Published by group.bmj.com.

7-7. https://www.cdc.gov/parasites/ strongyloides/epi.htm.

7-8. https://www.cdc.gov/parasites/ strongyloides/epi.html.

7-9. http://www.ivdresearch.com/strongyloides.php.

7-10. Parasitic worms and inflammatory diseases, P Zaccone,* Z Fehervari,* J M Phillips, D W Dunne, and A Cooke.

7-11. "...a few studies have shown that infection with helminth parasites can exaggerate existing disease, the consensus is that the generation of an immunoregulatory environment as a consequence of infection with parasitic helminths can reduce the severity of concomitant disease (an arrangement that would benefit parasites while they complete their lifecycle). "https://www.hindawi.com/journals/jpr/2011/942616/

8. VIRUSES

"I pictured myself as a virus...
and tried to sense what it would be like."

Jonas Salk

No doubt you're familiar with viruses, especially since it's highly unlikely you've reached adulthood without being affected by many of them. After all, they can cause everything from the annoyance of the common cold to illnesses that are life-threatening. And, they can cause arthritis.

However, you may also have heard that there are no drugs that are effective against them. While this is basically true, it doesn't mean there are no _remedies_ that are effective. Far from it. So no need to feel hopeless if you think your arthritis might have a viral cause. Instead, just read on. Learn how they operate so you're better equipped to use the list of remedies covered after the following brief explanation of their behavior. That way you'll be in a much better position to beat them at their own game.

Viruses are extremely tiny, especially considering the massive problems they can cause. (8-1) Viruses are composed of only two – or sometimes three - parts. All of them wear a protein coat on the outside that covers and protects their spiral shaped helix inside.

Some also have a viral wrapper – a fatty envelope that also encases them when they're not yet inside a cell. These 'envelopes' can actually fool your immune system into thinking they're not a threat. They do this so your immune system identifies them as being similar to other molecules that actually make up your body tissues, so your immune system doesn't attack them.

Viruses are extremely dependent little organisms. They can't actually live on their own, and they definitely can't replicate (make 'babies' - more like they are.) Instead, to live, grow and multiply, they depend on your own body cells. (8-2)

Viruses have a variety of ways to get into your joints and cause arthritis. Each virus has its own preferred method of transmitting itself. (8-3.) That said, there are six primary ways that viruses can infect you. They are:

1. exchange of blood,
2. exchange of body fluid by sexual activity,
3. oral exchange of saliva,
4. via contaminated food or water,
5. breathing in aerosol particles into your lungs that contain them, and
6. through animal or insect vectors such as mosquitoes.

There is also a 7th way viruses can get to your joints. You might notice it in particular if, say, you had an antibiotic treatment for a bacterial infection. Even if the antibiotic was effective in killing the bacteria, there's the fact that _viruses can live inside bacteria_.

This means that you could experience an arthritic flare-up after antibiotic treatment, because the bacteria the antibiotic killed was infected with a virus which is now directly exposed to your body tissues. These virus types – the ones that can infect bacteria are called 'bacteriophages'.

Rather than being unusual, such viruses - ones that can live in bacterial hosts are "one of the most abundant organisms on our planet; they are found in soil, ocean water, aerosols, and within animal intestinal tracts. Take, for example, the fact that " as many as 900 million viruses may occur in one milliliter of seawater, situated in surface microbial matting." (8-4)

They accomplish this by injecting their genetic material into the cell wall of the bacteria. The result: another cause of arthritis! (8-5)

So, now that you know _how_ some virus or other can manage to take up residence in your joints and cause arthritis, let's move on to the symptoms you might experience. Could you tell, based on your symptoms, for example, whether you had a viral or a bacterial joint infection?

The answer is, most likely, that the symptoms of viral infections of joints (as opposed to the bacterial ones mentioned before) are _milder_. Typically, you wouldn't even have a fever, but you might indeed ache all over. And no matter how many different antibiotics you took, they would not cure the problem. Additionally, such viral infections have the reputation of going away on their own. (8-6)

That said, sometimes what's true is that the symptoms _seem_ to have gone away, making you think the virus is gone too, only it emerges again later. It's as if these tiny little bugs were just taking a long nap.

Let's get down to some specific viruses that can cause arthritis. There are many that can do so, and the list is always changing. That's because the circumstances change in which they can hop on board. For example, arthritis caused by rubella (measles) is becoming less common, apparently due to vaccinations against it.

Meanwhile, other viruses depend on their carrier. These are called vector-borne transmissions, and are accomplished via the bite of some type of arthropod that's infected—bites from mosquitoes, ticks, triatomine bugs (blood suckers), sand flies, and black flies.

That said, on a worldwide basis, the following are just _some_ of the most common candidates for causing viral arthritis (in no particular order):

1. Influenza A virus (FLUAV)
2. Influenza B ((FLUBV)
3. Parvovirus b19,
4. Hepatitis B (HBV),
5. Hepatitis C (also referred to as HCV),
6. HIV (Human Immunodeficiency Virus)Type 1,
7. Ross River Virus (an alphavirus, a small, spherical, enveloped virus)
8. Sindbis virus (also an alpha virus)
9. Barmah forest virus (bfv) (an alpha virus)
10. Chikungunya infection
11. Natural RubellaIinfection,
12. Rubella immunization with RA 27/3 (Two live attenuated measles viruses in measles vaccines),
13. Hepatitis E
14. HTLV,
15. O'nyong-nyong fever
16. Mumps vaccination
17. Mumps polyarthritis
18. Epstein-Barr virus, and
19. Cytomegalovirus.

While it is unusual, other viruses, such as cytomegalovirus (CMV), herpes simplex virus (HSV) and varicella zoster virus (VZV) can cause arthritis – however, it is rare. (8-7)

Influenza virus: The influenza virus is probably the most commonly occurring of the three. Since you'd never be able to see it with your naked eye, take a look at it under an electron microscope:

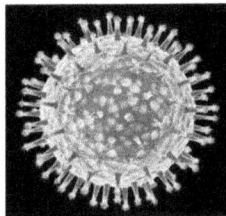

Figure 32 This is the viron that causes influenza.

Hepatitis C: The most common cause of viral hepatitis is the Hepatitis C virus. Hepatitis C virus (HCV) infection has been found to cause *rheumatoid arthritis*, even before HCV is detected. This is no casual infection, where you might feel punk for a few days and then recover: the Hepatitis C virus actually can contribute to liver failure.

Here's what it looks like:

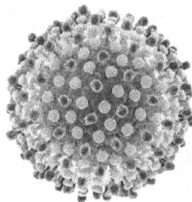

Figure 33 The Hepatitis C virus, one viral cause of arthritis.

Hepatitis B. This virus is the third most common cause of viral cause of arthritis. Here's what it looks like:

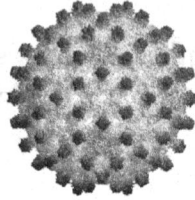

Figure 34 This Hepatitis B virus not only can cause arthritis; like it's cousin, Hepatitis C, it also is deadly.

❧

WHAT YOU CAN DO

So what can be done about viral infections of joints? Many medical doctors initially take the approach that a viral infection is self-limiting, and therefore, they do nothing about it. Therefore they may not offer any treatment directed at the virus itself, but rather at the symptoms.

Nonsteroidal anti-inflammatory drugs (NSAIDs) are the mainstay of treatment at this initial time. (8-8) (You can review the benefits and risks of these drugs in Chapter 2.)

If you are not satisfied with waiting six weeks, you may want to consider some herbal approaches, as these can be effective because they support your body's innate ability to fight viruses.

Doctors who follow the standard medical approach are unlikely to pursue further investigation unless the arthritis has persisted for more than six weeks. At that time, if they uncover Hepatitis B or Hepatitis C, they may initiate an aggressive approach aimed at strengthening your immune system response with such treatments as injections of 'interferons.' These are proteins your own body produces to fight infections, and a number of drugs have been created in the laboratory to mimic them. (8-9)

The action of another drug approach block the hepatitis C NS5B protein. (8-10) As of 2016, a 12-week course of treatment cost about US$84,000 in the United States, US$53,000 in the United Kingdom, US$45,000 in Canada, and US$483 in India. (8-9)

If you want to take advantage of the power of natural remedies, you'll be happy to know there are a number of them.

One of the easiest approaches for dealing with viruses has to do with strengthening your immune system so it can more easily rid your body of them. Below are some of the possibilities.

St. John's Wort is often effective against many (but not all) viruses that have an envelope structure. To review, an envelope virus is one that uses your own cell membrane to encase itself. These membranes become the outer fatty bilayer known as a viral envelope. The membrane is studded with proteins coded by the viral genome and host genome; the lipid (fat) membrane and any carbohydrates present are from your own cells. Both the Influenza virus and HIV virus use this strategy.

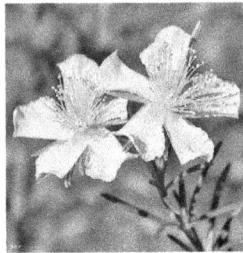

Figure 35 St. John's Wort

Echinacea can be helpful as it offers support for your immune system.

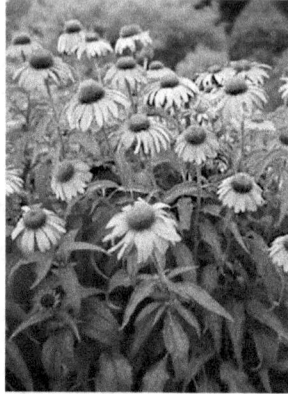

Figure 36 Echinacea purpurea

Astragalus is another herb that strengthens and tonifies your immune system.

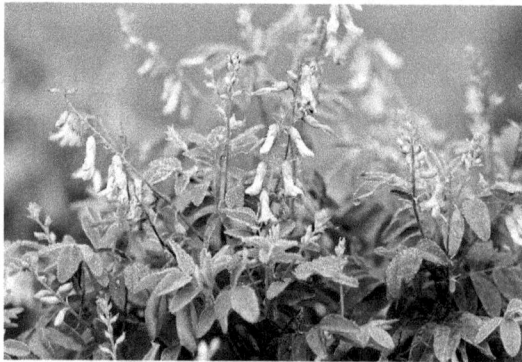

Figure 37 Astragalus

Ganoderma (also called Reishi, or Japanese Reishi) helps strengthen and improve your immune system functioning. It also supports your adrenal glands, (which are under stress during an infection), strengthens cell membranes and supports detoxification.

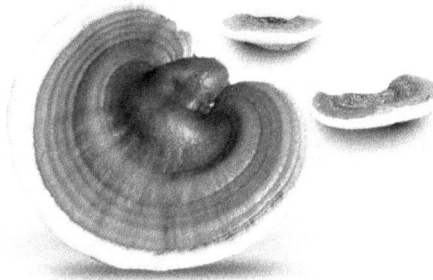

Figure 38 Ganoderma Lucidum mushroom

Sesame Seed Oil. If your virus is using a lot of your T cells (thrombocytes, a type of white blood cell), or if you want to support a higher T cell count so you can fight your infection better, you may benefit from Sesame Seed Oil. It contains the precursors your body uses to create thrombocytes. To get a sufficient amount of precursors, you may want to use a product that's been concentrated to provide them in higher amounts than you would get from, say, a teaspoon of sesame oil.

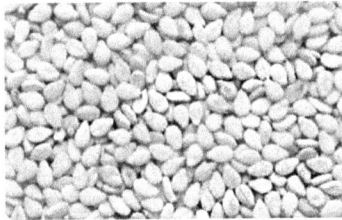

Figure 39 Sesame Seeds, from which the oil can be extracted.

Burdock Root is a blood purifier and lymphatic cleanser. It has also been shown to combat cancer cells by selectively stopping the proliferation of cancer cells and by inhibiting the cancer cells' production of particular proteins (NPAT proteins), hence crippling cancer's ability to reproduce.(8-11) Burdock root is an ingredient of many herbal combination products, and can also be purchased separately, often in liquid or tablet form.

73

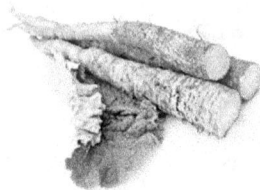

Figure 40 Burdock Root

Licorice and Echinacea together may prove to be an effective combination if you find your viral infection is hard to resolve. Other herbs and herbal combinations also exist. Rather than trying to make yourself into an herbalist, especially while under the duress of arthritic flare up, find an experienced health practitioner to guide you. (Check out resources for finding one in Chapter 18.)

***

Endnotes:

8-1. Most of them are only between 10 and 300 nanometers (nm). To give you an idea of how small that is, one nanometer is one *billionth* of a meter. Some of the larger ones – called filoviruses - can measure up to 1400 nm long with a diameter of approximately 80 nm http://eol.org/info/458

8-2. That's why one scientist (Rybicki) has portrayed them as operating "at the edge of life". That's also why viruses are differentiated as a totally separate form of life from other cellular organisms. E. P. Rybicki. 1990. The classification of organisms at the edge of life, or problems with virus systematics. S Aft J Sci 86:182–186 Advances in Virus Research RNA synthesis.

8-3. http://eol.org/info/458.

8-4. RNA synthesis. K. E. Wommack and R. R. Colwell. 2000.

Virioplankton: viruses in aquatic systems Microbiol. Mol. Biol. Rev. vol. 64, issue 1, pp 69–114.

8-5. Even though each bacteriophage is tiny in relation to the bacterial cell, nonetheless it can inject its genome inside the cell wall of bacteria. It does this first by rooting its long tail fibers into the cell wall , then it uses its tail structure to inject its genetic material through the bacterial cell wall. Drawn in part from C Michael Hogan (Lead Author); Sidney Draggan Ph.D. (Topic Editor) "Virus". In: Encyclopedia of Earth. Eds. Cutler J. Cleveland (Washington, D.C.: Environmental Information Coalition, National Council for Science and the Environment). [First published in the Encyclopedia of Earth May 12, 2010; Last revised Date December 30, 2010; Retrieved September 28, 2012. Encyclopedia of Earth.]

8-6. http://www.orthop.washington.edu/?q=patient-care/articles/arthritis/infectious-arthritis.html#causes.

8-7. Vassilopoulos d. Rheumatic manifestations of acute & chronic viral arthritis. In: imboden jb, hellmann db, stone jh, editors. Current diagnosis & treatment: rheumatology. 3rd edn. New york: mcgraw-hill; 2013.

8-8. https://www.racgp.org.au/afp/2013/november/viral-arthritis/

8-9. "Sovaldi 400 mg film coated tablets - Summary of Product Characteristics". UK Electronic Medicines Compendium. September 2016. Archived from the original on 10 November 2016. Retrieved 10 November 2016.

8-10. Hill, A; Simmons, B; Gotham, D; Fortunak, J (1 January 2016). "Rapid reductions in prices for generic sofosbuvir and daclatasvir to treat hepatitis C". Journal of virus eradication. 2 (1): 28–31. PMC 4946692 . PMID 27482432.

8-11. https://doi.org/10.1016/j.phymed.2013.08.003.

9. BACTERIAL INFECTIONS

Bacteria keeps us from heaven and puts us there.
Martin Fischer

If you have a negative association to the word 'bacteria', it's not surprising. It's easy to think of all bacteria as evil because some can make you sick. However, bacteria play a key role in not just your well-being, but your very survival.

For example, you wouldn't be able to digest your food without these living one-celled microorganisms: they help turn that meal you just ate into the nutrients and fuel you need to survive and thrive.

In fact, if some researchers are right, you might even owe the existence of your entire body to bacteria. They argue that the human body evolved as a collection of bacteria that learned to cooperate with each other, gradually developing into the collection of cells that make up the human body. (9-1)

All the bacteria living inside you right now would fill a half-gallon jug; the truth is you actually have 10 times more bacterial cells in your body than human cells. You actually have 30% _more_ bacteria in your body than you have human cells. (9-2)

Collectively, these colonies are referred to as your 'microbiome.' Most live in your gut, where they perform vital tasks, breaking down your meal into nutrient components your body can actually use to run and repair itself.

The fact is, if you were to manage to rid your body of all bacteria, you would no longer be able to live. Therefore the key to good health - and freedom from bacterial arthritis! - lies not in ridding your body of all bacteria, but rather in managing their colonies.

Of course, not all bacteria support your health. In fact, if you have joint inflammation due to an infection, the most likely culprit is some form of bacteria. The type of bacteria causing Lyme disease (covered in Chapter 6) is just one such bacteria — other types cause cholera, bubonic plague, rheumatic fever, meningitis and a host of other unpleasant, and even deadly illnesses.(9-3) That's the bad news.

The good news is, it's possible to selectively rid yourself of the ones that can cause you to become ill—and to do so without destroying the ones you need to be healthy.

❧

WHAT YOU CAN DO

Given how lethal these bacteria can be, you likely want to lower your risk, and happily, there are ways to do so. The first and most important is to avoid infection in the first place. The primary way to do that is revealed when you consider the role bacteria play in the larger ecosystem of the earth itself, where they play the vital role of recycling nutrients. To do so, they break down or decompose dead materials.

In other words, bacteria as a major biological species are responsible for the putrefaction stage in the process of turning dead or dying matter back into organic, living substances. This fact has major significance when it comes to preventing bacterial arthritis, or bacterial diseases of any kind.

Keep your body clean. It's crucial to keep your body clean, not only on the outside, but also on the inside. In other words, don't allow your body to become toxic. If you do, you're issuing a call for these bacterial invaders to come in and carry out their biological role. Keeping clean in the first place prevents the buildup of toxicity that requires their services to metabolize, or break it all down.

Ways to keep it clean include:

- drinking plenty of clean, pure water
- eating organic food free of pesticides
- making sure you completely digest the food you eat
- avoiding constipation

Keep good physical boundaries. When an invasion does take place, typically it does so through your skin or lungs or gut, and then travels through your bloodstream to your joints. To minimize this possibility, disinfect and protect any open skin wounds immediately until this breach in your outer boundary can heal.

A major way bacterial arthritis can begin is entry through your mouth. No doubt you're familiar with the all-too-common occurrence of food poisoning, causing a rapid evacuation of the offending bug via vomiting and diarrhea.

But your mouth can also be the origin of bacterial arthritis, especially if you have gum disease. In fact, if you have gum disease and even brush your teeth vigorously enough to break the 'skin' of your gums, you can end up with bacterial arthritis. That result is even more likely when you have dental work that interferes with the integrity of your gums, allowing pathogenic bacteria to enter your bloodstream. (9-4)

It also means taking care of leaky gut if that's an issue for you. (As there are different causes of leaky gut, and different remedies based on those causes, check with your health practitioner to help you sort it out.(9-5)

Pay attention to _early_ symptoms of bacterial joint inflammation. If bacteria do get an opportunity to take hold, the next strategy is to watch for early warning signs of joint inflammation.

General symptoms of bacterial joint inflammation happen quickly. That's because, under the best of conditions, certain bacteria "can grow and divide extremely rapidly, and bacterial populations can double as quickly as every 9.8 minutes." (9-6)

In addition to a sudden onset, watch for other general symptoms such as:

- Elevated body temperature
- Pain in the affected joint
- Swelling and redness
- Warm skin over the joint
- Lack of appetite
- Fatigue
- Elevated heart rate.

Ultimately, the type of bacteria causing your infection determine your symptoms. Your symptoms will also depend to some extent on your age. For example, children who have joint inflammation from a bacterial infection often complain of pain in their hips and shoulders, while as an adult, you will more likely experience joint pain from a bacterial infection in your arms or legs, and most especially in your knees.

If you're wondering how to know the whether your joint inflammation is due to bacteria or the previously discussed category of viruses, it is suggested that, "If the infection is bacterial (as opposed to viral), the pain is generally located in one place or area, it's usually accompanied by fever and shaking chills, usually begins quite suddenly." (9-7)

Medical tests available to determine You can take advantage of the following tests to help you decide your best course of action:

- Blood tests to detect the presence of harmful bacteria
- Joint X-ray to assess the extent of joint and cartilage damage
- Joint fluid sampling to determine the type of bacterial infection. (9-8)

The most likely culprits for causing bacterial arthritis (also called septic arthritis) are:

- Staph (from Staphylococcus aureus bacteria)
- Strep (from Streptococcal bacteria)
- Gonorrhea (from Neisseria gonorrhoeae bacteria)
- TB (Tuberculosis, from Mycobacterium tuberculosis)
- Lyme disease (from Borrelia burgdorferi, discussed in Chapter 6).

Let's take a closer look at four of these most likely culprits.

Staphylococcus Aureus (Staph Infections & MRSA*)* You've likely heard about staph infections, and for good reason. First of all, they naturally live on your skin–even if your skin is healthy (your skin microbiome). But, when they get virulent or when you get run down, they can pose a significant health risk.

Additionally, they've figured out how to evade the various antibiotics being thrown at them. These adapted staph bacteria are referred to as 'MRSA', which stands for 'Methicillin-resistant staph aureus.' Here's what they look like under a microscope in their characteristic clumping pattern:

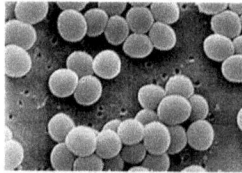

Figure 41 Don't be fooled by this pretty little colony—it's the potentially deadly Staph aureus, with its typical grape-like clusters.

While Staph infections can start on your skin, they can also travel to a joint from your sinuses. Or you might become infected as a result of surgery. If you were hospitalized, you're much more likely to pick up the type referred to as 'MRSA', (Methicillin resistant staph aureus). That's because most hospital staph bacteria have been sufficiently exposed to bactericides and antibiotics to have learned to outsmart them.

Additionally, you're much more susceptible to a staph infection if you have rheumatoid arthritis, if you take steroids or immunosuppressive agents (such as imuran, cytoxan and methotrexate) .

If you do become infected and the staph travels to your joint, your symptoms may include: fever, redness, swelling, extreme tenderness in a single joint, and possibly pus (yellowish-white substance) draining from a wound or abscess.

But make no mistake; if you experience the above symptoms *without* any other illness preceding it, staph or its smarter version, MRSA can still be the cause.

Streptococcus is a genus of bacteria whose name means ("twisted berry"), referring to its characteristic grouping in chains that resemble a string of beads. See here:

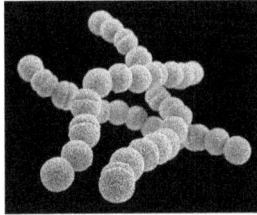

Figure 42 This streptococcus bacteria can be the culprit behind your arthritis.

Strep, as a family, has a large number of relations – different branches of the family tree that can be downright friendly or can cause all kinds of problems. The harmful ones are behind a great many cases of sore throats, ear infections, skin eruptions, some impetigo (others are from staph), scarlet fever and pneumonia, just to name a few.

One way strep can cause arthritis is actually a *response* to a strep infection. It's called 'reactive arthritis' or 'Reiter's Syndrome'. It's thought that the joint inflammatory reaction is a result of immune system activity. (9-9)

Strep bacteria can also cause arthritis when they get into your joint, causing rapid deterioration of its cartilage—even bone damage. Of course, this causes a great deal of pain and swelling, with redness around the affected joint. This type is called septic arthritis.

Strep arthritis is no lightweight problem; if not treated immediately and effectively, it can develop into some life-threatening and permanently damaging health problems including pneumonia, kidney damage, endocarditis (a heart infection) possibly cause your lungs to fail, not to mention permanent joint damage. The take-home message is to get an effective remedy immediately.

Medical treatment depends on the severity of the infection. It may involve antibiotics, sometimes administered intravenously, or might include draining the synovial fluid from the infected joint and immobilization of the joint to control pain. (9-10)

Neisseria gonorrhoeae or Gonococcus (gonorrhea) This is a bacterial infection transmitted via sexual contact – in fact it's one of the oldest known sexually transmitted diseases (STDs). It's also called 'the clap.' Because its spread between people by sexual contact, Prevent it with the correct use of condoms.

Here's what it looks like:

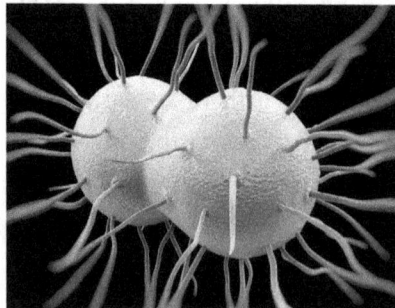

Figure 43 This bacteria is the cause of gonorrhea and gonococcal arthritis.

This bacteria is the cause of gonorrhea and gonococcal arthritis. Gonorrhea causes arthritis because these bacteria travel through your blood stream and can settle in one or more joints. Your knee joint is most commonly affected, but it can also attack your tendons and bursa to cause tendonitis and bursitis.

Infectious arthritis from gonorrhea can develop days or even weeks after the symptoms of gonorrhea appear. For some reason, it causes arthritis more often in women than in men. Its symptoms are easily mistaken for some other infection such as bladder infection. Also, its symptoms are not as obvious for women, which means women might seek treatment later after being infected than men. This delay in treatment gives the bacteria more time to travel through the bloodstream.

Symptoms of gonorrheal arthritis may include (9-11)

- No symptoms at all (more than half of infected women don't have symptoms)
- Fever
- Chills
- Abdominal pain in women
- Discharge from the penis or vagina (usually yellowish), sometimes vaginal bleeding
- Rash which appears as a few red rimmed dime-sized pus filled spots that are raised in the center
- Burning or frequent urination
- Genital redness or swelling
- With rectal gonorrhea infection–rectal discharge, anal itching, soreness and bleeding of the rectum and painful bowel movement.
- Inflammation of the tendons (bands that connect bones to muscles)
- Arthritis which develops in joints such as the knees or wrists.

If untreated, gonorrhea can lead to severe pelvic infections and even sterility. Complications in later life can include inflammation of the heart valves, arthritis and eye infections.

You should seek treatment as soon as you notice arthritic symptoms, because this type of arthritis can cause serious damage to your joints. Delaying in treatment gives the bacteria more time to travel through your bloodstream. Appropriate treatment with antibiotics can prevent damage to joints and other parts of your body. (9-12) In addition, it is suggested that if you have gonococcal arthritis, you should be treated for Chlamydia at the same time. (9-13)

Tuberculosis (mycobacterium tuberculosis) is a highly infectious and debilitating lung infection which can spread to your spine, your brain and also cause infectious arthritis. Happily, it is much less common today than it was years ago. When it does occur, it is often very slow to develop, and when it moves from your lungs to cause arthritis, it typically involves only one joint. Here's what the tuberculosis mycobacterium look like:

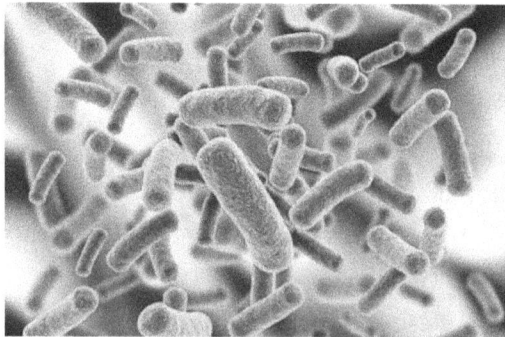

**Figure 44 This bacteria causes tuberculosis,
including tubercular arthritis.**

Tuberculosis, or TB, can be active or latent. Symptoms of the active tuberculosis lung infection, during which time you are infectious, include (9-14)

- Cough that lasts more than 3 weeks
- Chest pain
- Coughing up blood
- Feeling tired all the time
- Night sweats
- Chills
- Fever
- Loss of appetite
- Weight loss.

With the latent form of TB, you are carrying the bacteria, but your immune system is keeping it at bay until your resistance is sufficiently weakened that it can take over and become active. You are not infectious to others when your infection is latent.

Both forms are diagnosed using a chest x-ray, a skin test and blood tests. Long-term antibiotic therapy is employed over many months to treat the active phase. The latent phase may not be treated, but rather watched and not treated until it becomes active.

Non-antibiotic options. There are a number of non-antibiotic options that have been demonstrated to work for some bacterial infections. These include:

Goldenseal, an herb that contains particular phytochemicals (namely hydrastine and Berberine) with anti-bacterial properties. It also supports healing of mucus membranes – including those lining your digestive tract.

Garlic, long used in traditional medicine to help fight bacteria. The properties of the active compound in garlic, -Allicin has properties similar to penicillin. For best results, use it in its most potent form, which is raw and organic. A word of caution if you're taking blood thinning medications, however: garlic may interact with such drugs.

Aloe Vera has anti-microbial properties due to the polysaccharides in the gel of the inner leaves. They've been shown to activate several immune system components. You can consume aloe juice or take supplements that contain it.

Andrographus stimulates and supports your immune system functioning so it can fight off bacterial infections. Used for centuries in Chinese and other traditional medicine. (Note: don't use this if you're pregnant or breastfeeding, if you have myasthenia gravis, high blood pressure, heart or kidney conditions.)

Cinammon The essential oils in cinnamon both protect against bacterial infection and have anti-microbial properties that help fight it.

Echinacea has antibacterial properties, and enhances your immune system functioning, used for centuries to fight infections.

Olive Leaf contains many medicinally active compounds, among them oleuropein, which has demonstrated antibacterial properties.

If you're dealing with MRSA (Methicillin resistant staph aureus), your health practitioner might recommend you take a proteolytic enzyme on an empty stomach and follow that with an herb, such as Goldenseal, for example. The enzyme can break down the protein coat the 'smart' bugs use to evade your immune system, making them susceptible to both your immune system and to the herb.

Medical treatments for bacterial joint inflammation In general, these are treated with antibiotics after the bacterium causing the infection is identified. If your infection is more serious, you might receive antibiotics intravenously so the medication can flow directly into your bloodstream. Antibiotic treatment might take 2 to 6 weeks, depending on the type of bacterial infection you have and your overall medical condition. Your doctor might also drain the fluid around the joint to reduce pressure and eliminate harmful bacteria. (9-15)

Given the downstream serious effects that can result from these bacterial invaders, it's best to work with a qualified health practitioner and not try to solve it yourself. (See Chapter 18 if you need to find one.)

***

Endnotes:

9-1. Carolyn Bohach, a microbiologist at the University of Idaho (U.I.), along with other estimates from scientific studies, as quoted in Humans Carry More Bacterial Cells than Human Ones, Melinda Wenner, *The New York Times,*November 30, 2007.

9-2. Sender R, Fuchs S, Milo R (2016). "Revised estimates for the number of human and bacteria cells in the body". bioRxiv 036103.

9-3. http://www.orthop.washington.edu/?q=patient-care/articles/arthritis/ infectious-arthritis.html#causes)

9-4. https://en.wikipedia.org/wiki/Bacteria#cite_ref-101

9-5. Bacteria can also make you vulnerable to them. They do so by secreting chemicals into your bodily environment to modify it in their favor. Such secretions are often proteins acting as enzymes. That makes it possible for them to digest some form of what they consider to be food – actually to you they're toxins - they want to survive , multiply and thrive. http://www.drclark.net/disease-a-protocols/other-illnesses/arthritis

9-6. Eagon RG (1962). "Pseudomonas natriegens, a marine bacterium with a generation time of less than 10 minutes". Journal of Bacteriology. 83 (4): 736–7.

9-7. http://www.orthop.washington.edu/?q=patient-care/articles/arthritis/ infectious-arthritis.html#causes.

9-8. A fluid sample from your affected joint will change its appearance from its usual transparent thick quality. www.healthline.com/health/bacterial-joint-inflammation#diagnosis5

9-9. This form of arthritis " can last 3-12 months in the majority of patients. However, some patients can continue with symptoms beyond 12 months." Alan Matsumoto, M.D. https://www.hopkinsarthritis.org/ask-the-expert/strep-induced-arthritis/.

9-10. https://emedicine.medscape.com/article/236299-treatment.

9-11. https://www.stdrapidtestkits.com/blog/understanding-gonorrhea.

9-12. https://www.medicinenet.com/image-collection/the_clap_gonorrhea.htm.

9-13. https://emedicine.medscape.com/article/236299-treatment#d10

9-14 https://www.cdc.gov/tb/topic/basics/signsand symptoms.htm.

9-15. Often, this is done via arthroscopy. This procedure involves using tubes to drain and suction fluid. Arthrocentesis is another way to eliminate fluid. This procedure involves penetrating the joint area with a needle. In some cases, the joint must be irrigated and debrided. http://www.orthop.washington.edu/?q=patient-care/articles/arthritis/infectious-arthritis.html#basics.

10. YEAST, MOLD, CANDIDA: FUNGUS

Being challenged in life is inevitable,
being defeated is optional.

Roger Crawford

If you've heard anything at all about fungal infections, especially Candida, you've likely heard they are difficult to get rid of. But actually, they're not so tough to get rid of, they just need to be eliminated *slowly*. That's because killing them too rapidly can cause a die-off rate (or kill-rate) that's so fast it can overwhelm your body's elimination pathways, so you end up feeling much sicker than when you started.

So read on to discover the simple, procedural ways to both discover and gradually eliminate fungal infections. Once you understand their role in the ecosystem, you'll have a better grasp on how to address them effectively.

Fungi are actually a most interesting division of life. They're an entire separate category of life from plants and animals, yet they are just as significant. They include such subtypes as yeasts, molds and mushrooms.

Fungi are the principal decomposers in ecological systems both inside and outside your body. They live their lives pretty much under wraps – hardly detected unless they are fruiting. Then you might notice them as you might notice mushrooms or toadstools. (10-1)

By some estimates, fungi include, some 2.2 million to 3.8 million species, with only some 120,000 have been described as of this writing. Of these, eight thousand are detrimental to plants and 300 can be pathogenic to humans. Of these, the ones that happily invade your body and cause problems are those that grow well at mammalian body temperatures.(10-2) . Some of these that can cause disease, are the culprits behind fungal arthritis.

Together, they represent a huge variety of forms, some of them highly beneficial to people; others highly toxic and harmful. For example, they are highly prized as food when they exist in the form of mushrooms or truffles.

Some are sources of antibiotics , such as penicillin, which grows from bread mold. Others are used to make bread rise. Some – such as the yeast Saccharomyces cerevisiae, are used in baking, brewing and winemaking.

When you think of what they can do in your joints, consider the following two images. Think about how your joints would feel if the swelling (or 'proving') shown here were taking place in your joints instead of in a bowl:

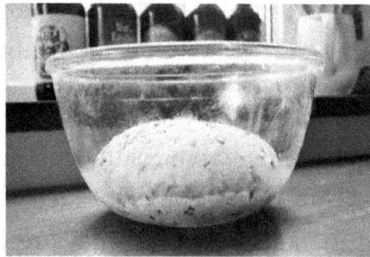

Figure 45 "Unproved" bread dough - no yeast!

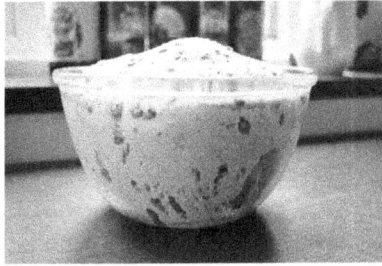
Figure 46 "Proved" bread dough -due to S. cerevisiae

What fungi do to your joints Although fungi are the least common infectious cause of arthritis, they're still significant enough to consider when tracing down the causes of your arthritis. If your arthritis is fungal, both your bone and also the soft tissue surrounding it - your entire joint - will be affected. This is most likely to take place in your knee, but that's not the only joint that can fungus can affect.

Are you susceptible? If you're healthy, you have a very low risk of developing fungal arthritis. That said, whether you are a man or woman, and regardless of your race or ethnicity or age, you can suffer from it. You may be especially susceptible if you are a gardener or a chicken farmer. That's because the particular types of fungi that can produce arthritis are usually found in soil, bird droppings and certain plants (especially roses). (10-3)

You arc definitely more at risk if you live or travel to or stay in areas when fungus is endemic, which is in warm, humid climatic conditions. You are especially susceptible if your immune system is weakened regardless of whether that's due to high stress, to hiv/aids, to cancer, to an organ transplant or even diabetes. You're also at greater risk if you're taking cortisone medication over time.

You are also more susceptible to any type of fungus if you are estrogen dominant. Fungi love an estrogen-rich environment. This may be why younger women have more fungal arthritis than younger men, - they have plenty of circulating estrogen, which drops as they age. But older men have more than older women as their estrogen levels increase with age. (10-4)

You can also get fungal arthritis if you're accidentally injected with medications from vials contaminated with fungal microbes. Sadly, this was exactly what happened when contaminated vials of medications produced by a compounding pharmacy caused a multistate outbreak of rare fungal meningitis and fungal arthritis in September 2012. (10-5)

If you've already been diagnosed with any of these following six fungal infections, you're also at an increased risk: (10-6)

- Blastomycosis
- Candidiasis
- Coccidioidomycosis
- Cryptococcosis
- Histoplasmosis
- Sporotrichosis

Rarely, fungal arthritis can also occur if a prosthesis used to replace a damaged joint was contaminated.

Regardless of why or how you got it, there are effective ways to address it.

༺ॐ༻

WHAT YOU CAN DO

Determine Fungus, Virus or Bacteria. First is to discover whether your arthritis is fungal as opposed to say, the bacteria or viruses we've already discussed. One way to tell is that arthritis produced by a fungus usually develops very slowly. That means the usual arthritic symptoms of pain, swelling, stiffness and redness of joints, with restricted range of motion also come on gradually. It might affect only one area or it can spread throughout your body. It may cause a low-grade fever, or you might have none at all, but bottom line, it begins quite slowly, developing over weeks or even months.

A closer look at two of the top causes of fungal arthritis will reveal the strategies that can eradicate it. First, Candida albicans, from the yeast lineage of the fungi family tree.

Candida albicans. There are two major reasons why candida albicans is a major player when it comes to fungal arthritis. First, is that candida is a normal part of the flora of your intestinal tract, which is not the problem. The difficulty arises from how tiny this one-celled organism is.

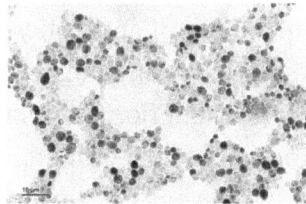

**Figure 47 Candida albicans, a yeast infection
that can produce arthritic symptoms.**

The cells that line your gut are about 1 micron apart if your gut is healthy. But, if anything happens to stress it—say you picked up a parasite, or you ate something that caused inflammation—the distance between the cells suddenly gets much wider, perhaps as much as 15 microns. To that tiny, one-cell wide Candida, that's a super highway. They happily move across, where they can now take up residence in your abdomen.

Now they're in an environment that's nutrient dense, it's richly oxygenated, it's dark, it's moist - what's not to like! The Candida starts having a party and making babies. Now it needs more sugar, which is what it thrives on, so it sends chemical signals to that part of your brain to make you crave carbohydrates.

Gradually, the Candida hijacks your nutrients, but most especially the oxygen your hemoglobin carries to go to your cells. The result is your cells slowly suffocate as the Candida takes over (a major reason systemic Candida infections cause so much fatigue). Perhaps that's one of the ways it becomes a precancerous condition. Research has demonstrated that Candida albicans can promote cancer by producing carcinogens, causing inflammation, increasing the response of Th17 cells, and molecular mimicry of your own immune cells. (10-7)

The second reason Candida comes in at the top of fungal arthritis causes has to do with the use of antibiotics. They may (or may not!) kill off some disease-causing bug, but in the process they also kill off part of the normal flora of your gut. That means less competition for nutrients, and the Candida thrives. Then with the stress and inflammation in your gut, they cross that boundary and they're _in._ Now they can easily set up residence in one of your joints.

Certain experiments have demonstrated this. A Dutch team in 2012 injected Candida albicans yeast cells into the knee joints of mice and found not only "joint swelling and inflammation", but also "enhanced destruction of cartilage and bone". (10-8)

Also, researchers at the University of Pittsburgh found that the presence of Candida caused an inflammatory response (specifically the production of TH17 cells). These are thought to play a role, not just in rheumatoid arthritis, but also other autoimmune diseases like psoriasis, multiple sclerosis, and Crohn's disease. (10-9)

Finding Out: The research studies above show a clear link between candida and arthritis. If you suffer from both of these conditions, beating your candida overgrowth can provide relief. If that sounds good, you can start by checking with a simple test you can do quite simply and easily yourself, and from the comfort of your own home.

Here's how:

- Do this in the morning, when you first get up, before you brush your teeth, and before have anything to eat or drink, not even water.
- Get a clear glass
- Fill it with water.
- Spit in the glass, and then don't disturb the water.
- If your saliva sinks to the bottom or forms stalactites or stalagmites (strings in the water) or if it forms globules suspended in the water, or 'cloudy' saliva that sinks, that's considered positive for Candida.
- If none of these things happen, don't move the glass, but recheck every 15 minutes or so for up to an hour. If none of these things has happened after an hour, you're considered to be clear of a systemic Candida infection.

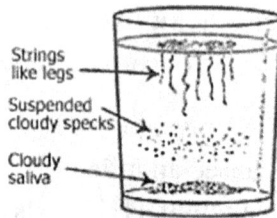

Figure 48 This simple home test can reveal your Candida status.

Then make sure you continue to have proper bowel flora and good pH, subjects we'll deal with in following chapters.

If your saliva test is not clear, you'll want to make a plan to address the problem. Attacking your candida will help with your arthritis in two ways. First, by destroying those candida colonies in your gut, you prevent the need for an inflammatory response from your immune system. Secondly, as you switch to a healthy, low-sugar eating plan to avoid feeding the fungus, you'll eliminate many of those pro-inflammatory foods from your diet too.

Prescription drugs. There are a variety of anti-Candida medications available by prescription. If you check their side effects and decide you don't want to go that route, you can work with a health practitioner that specializes in non-pharmaceutical approaches.

Non-pharmaceutical approaches. There are a number of effective herbal approaches to eliminating Candida. As they're also effective against mold, they're covered below.

Mold If you have a number of symptoms and can't seem to identify any cause, you might consider another member of the fungal family—something so tiny it's almost impossible to see—mold. An incredible variety of health problems—some of them seemingly unrelated—can have mucky mold at their root.

Molds, (sometimes spelled "moulds") are fungi that grow many-celled threads, or strands or filaments called hyphae. There are well over 100,00 identified types. Luckily only a few cause problems for people, but those few can cause big problems. (Others, penicillin, for example, are of considerable benefit.)

Mold loves environments rich in water, oxygen and nutrients along with a favorable temperatures, going dormant in temperatures below 40F or above 100F, and waiting until the temperature returns to their liking. Of course, your human body has all these qualities, which is why they're so happy to take up residence there.

They like dead organic material - another reason to keep your body as internally clean as possible. But they also like paper, wood and fabrics. They can even extract what they need to grow from some synthetics like adhesives or paints. Some molds can get enough moisture to grow from humid air (relative humidity above 70%).

Mold can enter your body through a wound or be inhaled into your lungs. Once inside, it starts growing by branching out from its tips (that 'hyphal growth'). It can reach your joints by travelling through your bloodstream.

Check this image below and you can imagine how a mold entering your lungs can cause major breathing problems once it starts branching out. As it grows, it invades blood vessels causing hemorrhages and death of tissue cells. If it continues growing, it can spread to other sites, such as your joints. Imagine what those branching structures can do once they enter your joint!

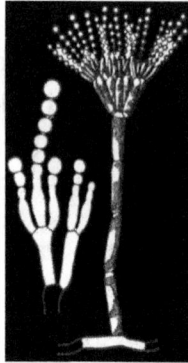

**Figure 49 note the way mold branches out—making it easy
to invade your tissues, including your joints.**

Some molds also cause illness by producing toxins—called
mycotoxins - that damage cell tissues. Some can also stimulate
your immune system, causing an allergic reaction. Over 200
different mold mycotoxins have been discovered, and some of
these substances are suspected of being able to cause DNA
damage. Some are so toxic that they were considered for
biological warfare agents in the 1940s. (10-10)

One of the most common, and most dangerous molds, is black
mold, or Stachybotrys. It's the stuff you might find in damp
corners of your house , because it thrives where materials have a
high cellulose content but low nitrogen such as paper, wallpaper,
drywall paper, fiberboard, gypsum board, particle board, seeds
and textiles.

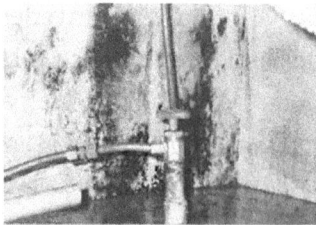

**Figure 50 Stachybotrys growing in a favorite place—
on sheetrock in a damp corner**

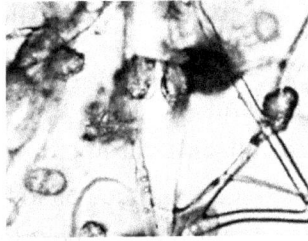

Figure 51 This is the all-too-common, and sometimes deadly, black mold, or Stachybotrys often found in houses, shown through a microscope.

It produces deadly mycotoxins which are airborne, and thus if you find such a problem in your house, _don't try to fix it yourself_. Instead, call a remediation specialist who can remove it with the correct equipment. (10-11)

If you suspect you may have a mold problem in your body, check to see if you have any of the following symptoms. For example, short term mold symptoms can include:

- Headache
- Shortness of breath, labored breathing.
- Unexplained bodily irritation, including rashes, itchy skin.
- Sensitivity to light.
- Runny nose, congestion, sinusitis.
- Coughing, throat congestion.
- Vision problems (eyes red, sore, dry, blurry or watery.
- Sneezing.

Long term symptoms can include:

- Tiredness, fatigue.
- Headaches, migraine.
- Achiness, pains or fever (including in ears, sinuses, joints

and muscles, swollen glands) or other symptoms of infection.

- Breathing problems, including wheezing, shortness of breath, asthma attacks, chronic bronchitis.
- Neurological symptoms such as loss of short or long term memory, speech problems, unexplained changes in personality and mood.
- Nose bleeds.
- Coughing up blood or blackish debris.
- Loss of appetite, nausea, vomiting, weight loss, diarrhea.
- Hair loss.
- Skin rashes, open skin sores.

Without effective treatment, you may develop symptoms severe enough to prevent you carrying out your usual daily activities. Your joint damage may advance to the point where you can't even carry out your usual daily activities. In short, not recommended! To avoid that fate, address it as early as you discover it. That way you stand the best chance of preventing it from getting to your joints.

Pharmaceutical Drugs. Diagnosing a mold infection is a medical challenge, arrived at with a combination of laboratory tests and symptoms. If you seek medical diagnosis, you will be given an evaluation of your medical history and physical exam, including your joints. Your physician may look for redness, swelling, and warmth of the joint, as well its range of motion. You may have the synovial fluid aspirated so it can be examined under a microscope by pathologist, which is how a definitive diagnosis can be made. You may also receive an X-rays of your joint, and a blood test to check for positive antibodies.

If they decide mold is the culprit, you will likely be prescribed an antifungal drug. The drug choice will be based on the particular mold that is suspected or was isolated from tests. The medication Amphotericin b is one such possibility.

If your joint involvement is severe, surgery may be required to remove the infected tissue.

Before considering the options below, know that fungal arthritis is considered a medical emergency that requires immediate treatment.

Non- Prescription Choices. For non-medical emergencies, practitioners employing a non-pharmaceutical approach to ridding the body of mold or Candida may use digestive enzymes. Here's how it works: You take digestive enzymes, only instead of taking them with meals, which would aid your food digestion, you take the recommended enzymes on an empty stomach. That allows them to get past your digestive system. When they enter your circulation, they can come in contact with the growing ends of the strands or filaments (remember those hypha?) and the exoenzymes and digest them.

If you are having allergic symptoms caused by mold, you may have various homeopathic remedies recommended to you, such as Allium Cepa, butterbur and biminne.

Your natural medicine practitioner (see Chapter 18 for finding these practitioners) might recommend among the following for addressing either Candida or mold that's not a medical emergency:

Methods to support your body's own defenses in dealing with fungi. These center on adapting your internal environment to be one that does not favor fungal growth. They include dietary changes such as reducing dairy products, sugars, including honey and fruit juice, and foods like beer that contain yeast, consuming mainly uncooked and unprocessed foods and adding fermented foods and/or probiotics.

They also might point out something it may be difficult to believe. Your cell phone, microwave or smart meter might be contributing to the progression of your arthritis. This is entirely possible because funguses thrive on electromagnetic frequencies, or emf's.

Cat's Claw contains seven different medicinally active alkaloids that increase the body's immune response. Used for over 2000 years by South American tribes.

Oregano Oil is effective against Candida because it contains Carvacrol, which has powerful antimicrobial properties. Like Grapefruit seed extract (below) it's been shown to help break through the Candida's outer cell membranes.

Garlic, discussed in the previous chapter, has many sulfur-containing compounds that help fight Candida.

Grapefruit Seed Extract is a potent antifungal agent. It has the added advantage of containing many bioflavonoids and antioxidants. It breaks down Candida's cell walls. It also gives a boost to your immune system.

Myrrh has strong anti-fungal properties, but don't use it if you're taking anticoagulants. (10-12)

Whichever remedy you employ, go slowly. You don't want to deal with a high kill-rate and make yourself really sick!

After the mold seems to be cleaned up – both in your body and in your environment, the next task at hand is to repair the tissue involved. For this a combination of herbs and nutrients are available.

Health practitioners have employed these strategies with good results, so be reassured. Even though you might have a mold problem in your body, you don't have to keep having it!

***

Endnotes:

10-1. Fungi can grow in association with other plants, as when they associate with algae to form lichens. https://en.oxforddictionaries.com/definition /fungus.

10-2. Fems yeast res. 2006 jun;6(4):463-8.

10-3. http://www.orthop.washington.edu/?Q=patient-care/articles/arthritis/infectious

10-4. Ibid.

10-5. Carol A. Kauffman, M.D., Peter G. Pappas, M.D., and Thomas F. Patterson, M.D.N Engl J Med 2013; 368:2495-2500June 27, 2013DOl: 10.1056/NEJ Mra1212617

10-6. According to http://www.orthop.washington.edu/?Q =patient-care/articles/arthritis/infectious-arthritis.html #causes

10-7. http://library.med.nyu.edu/cgi-bin/Shibboleth_ezp_ds.pl? entityD=NYULMCezpProdEntityID&return=https%3a%2f%2fl ogin.ezproxy.med.nyu.edu.

10-8. This study concluded that "minute amounts of fungal components, like C. albicans, are very potent in interfering with the local cytokine environment in an arthritic joint, thereby polarizing arthritis towards a more destructive phenotype." Marijnissen RJ, Koenders MI, van de Veerdonk FL, Dulos J, Netea MG, Boots AM.

10-9. Arturo casadevall, liise-anne pirofski Immunoglobulins in defense, pathogenesis, and therapy of fungal diseases Cell host & microbe, volume 11, issue 5, 17 may 2012, pages 447-456.

10-10. http://drjaydavidson.com/toxic-mold-lyme/.

10-11. https://www.mold-advisor.com/mycotoxins-and-joint-pain.html .

10-12. https://www.medicinenet.com/fungal_arthritis/article.htm#what_causes_fungal_arthritis.

11. MICROBIOME DISTURBANCES

The future depends on what we do in the present.
Mahatma Ghandi

The bugs in your tummy play a major role in whether or not you'll develop arthritis. That's really good news, because it means you can adjust them with the possibility of impacting your arthritis in a positive way.

To understand how that's possible, and gain some insight knowing what to do and not do, here's a closer look at where these bugs - collectively referred to as your 'microbiome' - actually come from and their role in your health, especially that of your joints.

The bugs that make up your intestinal flora have existed in humans as long as humans have existed. However, they did _not_ exist _in you_ to begin with. Instead, you inherited the first ones that began to inhabit your gut from your mother during your prenatal development and birth process.

If you were delivered via C-section, or your mother got antibiotics during your delivery, you missed out on some or all of this inheritance. The significance of this fact is just beginning to be understood and appreciated – including its importance in the development of arthritis. (11-1)

The result is that by the time you became an adult, your human biome contained—and still contains—trillions of bacteria. Here are some of the factors that go in to the makeup of your microbiome as it evolves over the course of your life.

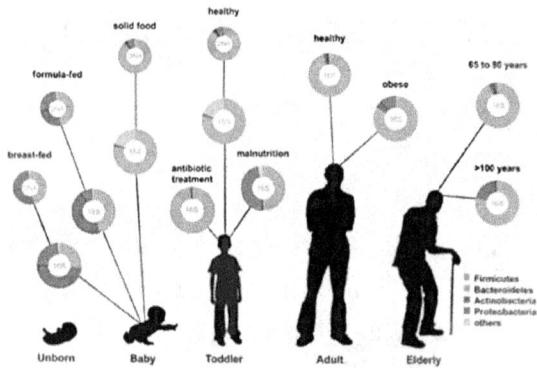

Figure 52 The characteristics of human microbiota change over time in response to varying environmental conditions and life stages.

As you can see, the changes that take place while you're going through life's stages also modify your unique microbiome which is so crucially important to your survival and thriving.

You likely know that your *genetic* inheritance functions like a blueprint or set of instructions for making and repairing all parts of your body. What has been less known until recently is that your *microbiotic* inheritance overlays that genetic blueprint where it: (11-2)

- Becomes a source of genetic diversity
- Can help modify any disease you might experience
- Becomes an essential component of your immunity
- Influences your metabolism
- Adjusts your interactions with drugs

These are just some of the reasons why it's referred to as your 'second genome'. But that's not all these flora do for you. They also do the following:

- Ferment your intestinal contents
- Train your immune system

- Help you contain other unwanted flora such as pathogens or opportunists
- Regulate your gut development
- Help recirculate bile acids
- Produce beneficial vitamins such as biotin and vitamin K,
- Manufacture hormones that affect your fat storage

That describes just some of their role in your health status. What they get in return, is to be able to thrive in a nutrient-rich, protected environment – your gut. (11-3)

Your Gut Microbiome and Arthritis. The first way your gut flora can set you up for arthritis has to do with the fact that 80% of your immune function is located in your gut. You have 'Peyer's patches', that line the lower part of your small intestine. These are small patches of lymph tissue that serve a special and significant purpose—they are an initial layer of defense against pathogens.

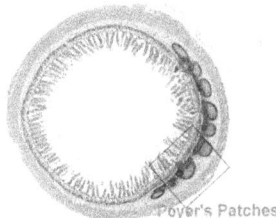

Figure 53 If you could look down the 'tube' of your small intestine, you would find Peyer's patches in the lining all around it.

Damage to the lining. With good intestinal barrier function, your intestines are protected from toxins and harmful microorganisms, yet nutrients are allowed to pass into your system. Anything that inflames or damages your small intestine can negatively affect this layer of defense, setting the stage for pathogens and toxins to enter, possibly arriving at your joints.

And it all starts with inflammation.

That's an overview of how the microbiome in your gut can cause arthritis in your joints. Here are some specifics for how that damaging gut inflammation can get set up and what you can do about it.

❧

WHAT YOU CAN DO

Eliminate Food Intolerances. You may recall this subject from Chapter 3: having a food intolerance means your body can't completely digest a particular food. Based on clinical evidence, many health practitioners say the # 1 cause of gut inflammation is inability to digest wheat!

When you eat wheat, the normal space between one gut cell and another, - only one micron - gets expanded to 15 microns. This is akin to creating a superhighway for all manner of yuk to cross over into your body. What this implies is that the #1 strategy for eliminating gut inflammation is to eliminate wheat from your diet. But don't panic! - you can still have rye, buckwheat, barley, millet, oats etc.

However if you're gluten intolerant, you'll need to limit your grain consumption to these four basic gluten-free grains: rice, millet, amaranth, quinoa. Failing to do so can have your gut looking like this:

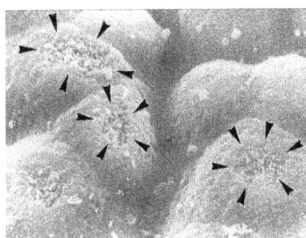

Figure 54 This image shows gut lining damage caused by exposure to gluten in a gluten-sensitive person.

Eliminating gluten—or even just wheat—is not a straightforward task, given that wheat is present in so many foods and products. Sometimes it's even used as a filler in nutritional supplements and prescription drugs. You will need to make a habit of asking your pharmacist to review the drug database of any pharmaceutical for hidden elements of wheat or gluten.

Nonetheless, it can be done, as many people who are gluten intolerant can tell you, and it's not as difficult as it may seem at first. You can start by first becoming aware of the sources of wheat you're consuming, and then gradually work to eliminate them.

It's just one step, but one that many people have discovered corrects their gut symptoms completely. And some who have made this change (not all, but some) have noted that they shed a number of unwanted pounds as well, without even thinking about it. Those are huge health benefits from making one simple change!

Of course, there are many other food intolerances. Lactose intolerance is another common one–apparently 98% of Asian adults and over 50% of non-Asian adults are lactose intolerant. Your particular genetics determine some specific foods your body won't be able to digest. You can find a list of these according to your blood type, at www.4yourtype.com.

Metals can also set up gut inflammation. The most common sources of metals getting into your gut are from eating contaminated food (seafood containing mercury, for example) or dental amalgam fillings that leak mercury. You can find a resource on metal toxicity, where it comes from and how to detox safely at www.freeoftoxicmetals.com.

Chemicals can set up intestinal inflammation. A common source of these is the pesticide residue on non-organic food. Eliminating this source by consuming organic food only can allow your body to resolve this source of inflammation.

Intestinal toxicity can arise from something as simple as eating a food you can't completely digest. Over time, the contents sit in your gut where they putrefy, and, as pointed out previously, the role of bacteria in any ecosystem – including your gut – is to break down decaying matter. There are a number of products on the market to help you deal with this. A great place to start is to increase your fiber intake through your diet. You can also find a dietary fiber supplement that agrees with you.

Gut dysbiosis means your gut flora contains too few beneficial bacteria, a result of being crowded out by an overgrowth of harmful pathogens, such as bacteria, yeast, even parasites. You may have heard of a couple of these - Clostridium difficile (C.diff) and Pseudomonas (not good When this happens, your intestinal microbes switch from maintaining your gut health to promoting inflammation." (11-4) The downstream result can manifest arthritis. In this situation, instead of producing health, your microbiome, with its over-colonization with pathogens, produces disease. (11-5)

This has been scientifically demonstrated: particular genes operating in association with your gut microbiome can determine your immune environment, and that in turn can result in your becoming susceptible to arthritis. (11-6)

One of the primary causes of dysbiosis is turning out to be genetically modified foods (GMOs). Several studies have shown that the organisms (mostly bacteria) of the microbiome can take up genes from GMO foods. (11-7). "Conjugation", or gene transfer, is a common trick used by bacteria to evolve and adapt. This is one mechanism by which antibiotic resistance perpetuates. (11-8)

There are a variety of supplement products that can help with this. For example, probiotics products help swing your microbiota balance back toward the more friendly bacteria. Particular herbs can render your gut an unfriendly place for pathogens. Still others work to rid your body of GMO's, taken in conjunction with consuming only organic foods and supplements.

Leaky gut As stated before, the ability of your microbiome to either set you up for arthritis or protect you from it has to do with its ability to cause or to prevent inflammation. Intestinal inflammation sets the stage for 'leaky gut', a condition that starts when the lining of your intestine has become too permeable. In other words, its leaking food particles and the stuff that's supposed to go down and out, which starts oozing into your belly. Here's how it progresses from a leaky gut all the way to autoimmune arthritis:

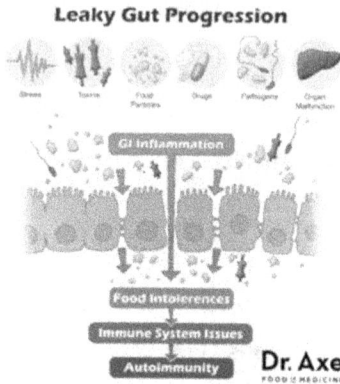

Leaky Gut Progression

Figure 55 This chart shows just how severe the downstream effects
of leaky gut can become if allowed to continue.

Since leaky gut is so significant an issue, you can check the
following symptoms to make some guesses yourself about the
condition of your gut:

- You may experience only vague symptoms initially,
  like feeling a little bloated and gassy, as if you ate
  too much, even though you know you didn't. (That's
  due to inflammation.)
- You might feel a vague discomfort in your belly—
  like a general achiness. (That's due to an
  inflammatory reaction too.)
- You may come down with colds and flu more easily
  than you had. (That's because so much (80%!) of
  immune function is located in your gut.)
- You might notice more and more foods give you
  problems. (That's because those undigested food
  particles are now circulating around where your
  immune system identifies them as foreign proteins,
  which they are, and attacks them).

- You might have unexplained dull headaches and bouts of fatigue.
- Sometimes you might even have cramps in your intestine, and think you ate something that didn't agree with you. In that part, you might well be right.

If you notice such symptoms, you can work with a qualified health practitioner who can make recommendations for you to heal it. One such suggestion is likely to be to eat more broccoli, because recent studies have demonstrated it's good for your gut. Brussels sprouts and cauliflower may also have these gut-health promoting properties. The study concluded the amount necessary would be around 3.5 cups of broccoli each day or a cup of Brussels sprouts. (11-9)

Last, you can also get your gut microbiota analyzed by a laboratory. Here is a comparison of two forms that can take. (Other companies can be found online.)

16S Sequencing	Viome Metatranscriptome Sequencing
Identifies only a fraction of your gut bacteria; unable to identify nonbacterial microorganisms	Identifies all bacteria and all other living organisms in your gut: viruses, archaea, yeast, fungi, parasites, and bacteriophages[5]
Low resolution (genus level only)	High resolution (species & strain level)
Does not determine microbe function	Quantifies the biochemical activities of all gut microorganisms
Unreliable; sequencing the same sample twice can yield very different results[3]	Unbiased analysis, minimized variation in results
Unable to identify microbial metabolites, which are key for maintaining health	Identifies which metabolites are being produced and which are missing
Low resolution and lack of functional data preclude any actionable recommendations	Allows correlation of microbes and their functions with common chronic conditions, so actionable recommendations can be made

Figure 56 This is one example of one at-home testing method and what it can reveal about your particular microbiome.

Your gut microbiota influences all your intestinal immune responses during both health and disease. Keeping it balanced and healthy is a major key to not just preventing or resolving arthritis, but also a host of other diseases.

***

Endnotes:

11-1. Until you were born, you were encased in your mother's womb - an environment completely free of any microorganisms. Then, during birth and after, you were exposed to the microbes from your environment. These competed for dominance, and by your first birthday, the various bugs that now make up your adult microbiome were established – often a thousand or more types. Dominguez-Bello MG, et al. Delivery mode shapes the acquisition and structure of the initial microbiota across multiple body habitats in newborns. Proc. Natl acad. Sci. Usa. 2010;107:11971–11975.

11-2. annu rev genomics hum genet. 2012; 13: 151–170.

11-3. Http://teca.fao.org/sites/default/files/comments/ files/gmo%2cshikimate _pathway_gut_flora_ and_health.pdf.

11-4. Round jl, mazmanian sknat rev immunol. 2009 may; 9(5):313-23.

11-5. http://teca.fao.org/sites/default/files/comments/ files/GMO%2CShikimate_pathway_gut_flora_and_health.pdf

11-6. Gomez a, luckey d, yeoman cj, marietta ev, berg miller me, murray ja, et al. (2012) loss of sex and age driven differences in the gut microbiome characterize arthritis-susceptible *0401 mice but

not arthritis-resistant *0402 mice. Plos one 7(4): e36095.
https://doi.org/10.1371/journal.pone.0036095

11-7. Carl-Alfred Alpert, Denis D G Mater, Marie-Claude Muller, Marie-France Ouriet, Yvonne Duval-Iflah, Gérard Corthier. Worst-case scenarios for horizontal gene transfer from Lactococcus lactis carrying heterologous genes to Enterococcus faecalis in the digestive tract of gnotobiotic mice. Environ Biosafety Res. 2003 Jul-Sep;2(3):173-80.

11-8. M Gruzza, M Fons, M F Ouriet, Y Duval-Iflah, R Ducluzeau. Study of gene transfer in vitro and in the digestive tract of gnotobiotic mice from Lactococcus lactis strains to various strains belonging to human intestinal flora. Microb Releases. 1994 Jul;2(4):183-9.

11-9. Gary Perdew, Ph.D, https://www.sciencedaily.com/ releases/2017/10/171012151754.htm.

12. GENERALIZED ACIDITY

In the middle of every difficulty lies opportunity.

When you're already suffering with joint pain, you can feel it's really unfair when you have other strange symptoms along with it. Yet that can be a blessing in disguise: considering them as a package can show you the common root hiding their resolution.

Arthritis can be brought into being by states that are too acidic, a bodily state that has other seemingly unrelated symptoms. Happily, all of them resolve together when this is corrected.

Your body is designed so that all its various processes run best when its fluids are not too acidic and not too alkaline. The scale used to express this state is called 'pH'. In practical terms, pH refers to the relative acidity or alkalinity of any of these bodily fluids – saliva, blood, urine, lymph etc.

The term itself refers to the relative concentration of hydrogen ions. They are expressed on a scale from 0 to 14. The low numbers express acidic states, while higher numbers convey alkaline states. The middle of the scale, 7, refers to a neutral state.

The following image illustrates some pH readings for various liquids.

pH scale*
*approximate pH numbers

| 0 | 1 | 2 | 3 | 4 | 5 | 6 | 7 | 8 | 9 | 10 | 11 | 12 | 13 | 14 |

hydrochloric acid — upset stomach acid — normal stomach acid — lemons — battery acid — sodas — vinegar — acidic soil — orange juice — tomatoes — bananas — coffee — salmon — potatoes — normal rain — bread — milk — human saliva — blood — pure water — seawater — phosphate detergents — eggs — baking soda — antacids — borax — milk of magnesia — ammonia — nonphosphate detergents — bleach — sodium hydroxide

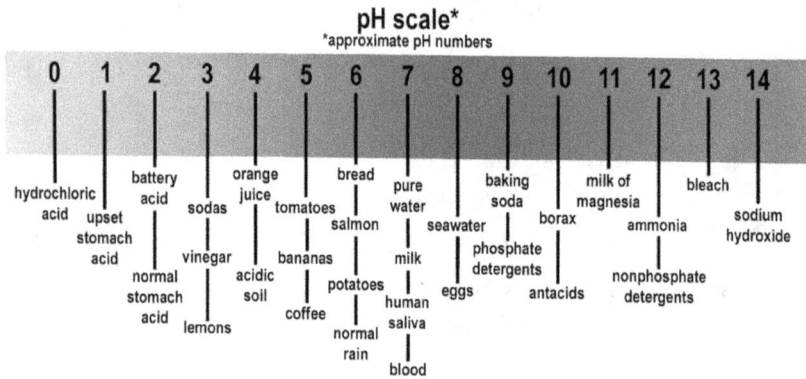

Figure 57 Various substances and bodily fluids have different pH readings.

Like other living things, your body depends on the right pH levels to keep you alive and thriving. Each of your bodily fluids - saliva, blood, urine etc. not only has a pH, it has its own _optimal_ pH. For example, blood flowing through your veins requires a pH between 7.35 and 7.45.

In general, any bodily tissues that come in contact with the external environment need an acid pH to function well. Bodily fluid _outside_ your cells, such as blood plasma and interstitial fluid want an alkaline pH. Fluid _inside_ your cells want a slightly alkaline pH. Although different sources state slightly different numbers considered in the normal range, these numbers are still relatively close to each other. Here is one such estimation: (12-1)

Gastric acid (your stomach acid) 1.25-3.0
Urine 6
Muscle Intracellular Fluids 6.1
Saliva   6.35-6.85
Liver Intracellular Fluids 6.9

Blood Plasma   7.4
Pancreatic Juice   7.8-8.0

If your blood exceeds its necessary pH range by as little as one-tenth of a pH unit, that could prove fatal! That's why, if these ranges are off, even slightly, your body uses some of its built-in buffering mechanisms correct it. Keeping the relative pH within that optimal functioning range is crucial. Since arthritis is brought about by acidic states, it's worth delving deeper into how your body attempts to deal with it.

Your body uses water or other alkaline fluids to neutralize too much acidity. It pulls bicarbonate from your pancreas into your blood to counter the acid. It filters acidic agents out through your skin, lungs or urinary tract (which accounts for certain body odors).

In fact, any pH states that are too low (acidic), and within nanoseconds, your body grabs calcium and magnesium ions out of your bones or teeth (a major contribution to osteoporosis). In less time than a heartbeat, it averts a pH state that's heading out of balance and brings it back to a more neutral, life-supporting and life-sustaining state.

Your body has one more remedy for high acidity, and that also results in arthritis: it can deposit acid substances into your joints. Those farthest away from your vital organs (your heart and lungs) are its first choice – meaning that you'll develop arthritis in your wrists, finger joints and, toe joints. This is its last option – if the acidic state continues, cells begin to die and ultimately you die too. (12-2)

As outlined above, what this means in terms of arthritis is that the ongoing acidity can etch away the lining of your joints, resulting in an inflammatory arthritis. Not only is a proper, well-balanced pH, not too acid, not too alkaline, highly protective of your health, it also makes it difficult for health problems to occur.

These are just some of the reasons health practitioners pay careful attention to the pH of your various bodily fluids.

§

WHAT YOU CAN DO

To aim for diminishing or even eliminating joint pain and the various weird symptoms that go along with an acid pH, you'll need to know which numbers you should use to assess whether or not your pH is in balance.

As different areas of your body function best at different pH readings, each bodily fluid you test has its own specific optimum pH range.

The most important pH is your intracellular fluid, because keeping it neutral is how metabolites (intermediate products of metabolism, or breakdown of food) are all charged and kept inside your cells where they're needed. To heal arthritis, you'll need a slightly alkaline intracellular fluid. Getting and keeping this pH into the slightly alkaline range is fundamental to any effective health-improving strategy, but especially one involving arthritis.

However, intracellular pH isn't the only important number. The pH of your digestive tract is also vital. That's because particular pH values are required to extract nutrients from the food you eat. Each digestive area has its own optimal pH.

The following are generally accepted ranges for areas of your digestive tract:

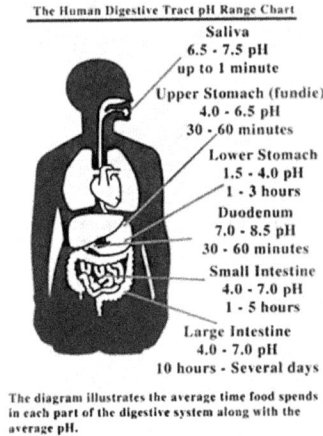

The Human Digestive Tract pH Range Chart

Saliva
6.5 - 7.5 pH
up to 1 minute

Upper Stomach (fundie)
4.0 - 6.5 pH
30 - 60 minutes

Lower Stomach
1.5 - 4.0 pH
1 - 3 hours

Duodenum
7.0 - 8.5 pH
30 - 60 minutes

Small Intestine
4.0 - 7.0 pH
1 - 5 hours

Large Intestine
4.0 - 7.0 pH
10 hours - Several days

The diagram illustrates the average time food spends in each part of the digestive system along with the average pH.

Figure 58 This is one estimate of the pH values needed for healthy digestion.

How you can tell if your pH is off: Checking your symptoms.
Use the following list to acquaint yourself with symptoms of pH that's too low or too high, and find out how many apply to you. Remember they can change from one time to another, so don't assume they'll be the same in, say, a week, as they are now. Also remember that you might not have any; so use other methods as well.

The following are among the symptoms of a pH that's too high:
(12-3)

Common metabolic alkalosis symptoms (too high a pH)

- Feeling light-headed
- Confusion
- Nausea
- Vomiting
- Hand tremors
- Involuntary muscle twitching
- Sensations of numbness or tingling in the face, arms or legs
- Hypersensitive reflexes
- Cramping
- Prolonged and involuntary muscle spasms, particularly in the hands and feet
- Catatonic stupor
- Coma
- Shock
- Ultimately death.

These symptoms are those of a pH that's too low: (12-4)

Common metabolic acidosis symptoms (too low a pH)

- Fatigue or drowsiness
- Becoming tired easily
- Confusion
- Shortness of breath
- Sleepiness
- Headache

How you can tell if your pH is off:
Checking your own pH.

You can get pH strips to use to take your own pH readings. You'll find a number of kits for self-testing pH kits online or at your local pharmacy. When you test yourself, you'll be asked to compare the test strip you've infused with your own bodily fluid with a scale that looks like this:

THE PH SCALE

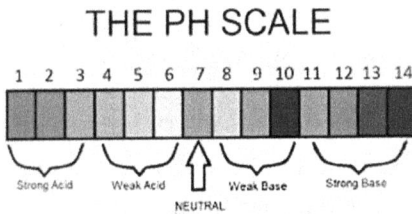

Figure 59 Strong acids are represented by the lower numbers; strong bases (alkalis) by higher numbers.

Follow the directions on the package for how to use them for each bodily fluid you're checking. Then, too, remember that the normal values for one fluid, say, saliva, are very different from those for normal urinary pH. Also, if you're receiving a blood test, you can ask the person ordering it to make certain that pH is reported along with other results.

Remember that the **most important pH to check for arthritis is the _intracellular_ one** because **those fluids affect joints most directly. This pH is reflected in your _saliva_.** The **second** most important one is your **urinary pH.** You won't be able to check your blood pH unless you prick your skin, and that's really not necessary to get the information you need.

If not corrected, low pH levels can lead to arthritis, kidney problems, kidney stones, kidney failure, plus bone problems.

Now that you know how important pH is, let's consider how to positively affect your own pH.

Correcting your pH

Dietary corrections: Paying attention to your diet is key in returning your pH back into the normal range. This is especially significant for people consuming the typical Western diet because it's acid forming, loaded as it is with meats, cheese and processed grains. In addition, it's also low in alkaline forming foods like fruits and vegetables.

What goes into your body has everything to do with its pH after digestion. That said, it's important to remember that getting the pH-altering effect you desire from any food is the pH it has *after* you have digested it. Therefore, various charts about the pH of any particular food *before* you digest it are of little consequence.

Reduce intake of acid-forming foods. To encourage your body to return to its optimal pH, reduce eating acid-forming foods. These include:
- processed meats and cereals
- high sodium foods
- fried foods
- refined grains
- coffee
- alcohol.

Increase intake of alkaline forming foods, such as:
- Plant proteins
- Dark, leafy greens
- Starchy plants
- Most fruits

Eat a good percentage of them raw, or only lightly steamed.

Increase intake of pH balanced foods. The most balancing food to eat is brown rice. Algaes and grasses are also pH balanced, in addition to being nutrient dense and mineral rich. Spirulina, kelp and wakame are among the choices.

Use apple cider vinegar. A common folk remedy for correcting pH (and a number of other health issues) is apple cider vinegar. In certain individuals, it can help restore proper pH balance. If you're not sure if it's for you, or you just don't like how it tastes, you might consider using it in a detox bath.

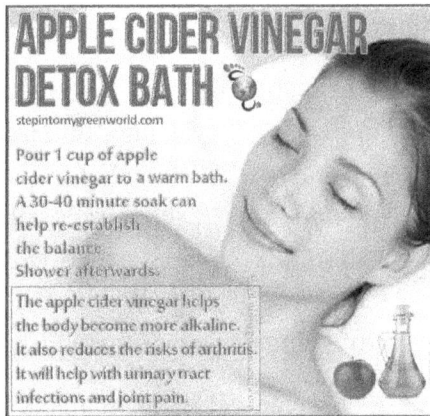

APPLE CIDER VINEGAR DETOX BATH

stepintomygreenworld.com

Pour 1 cup of apple cider vinegar to a warm bath. A 30-40 minute soak can help re-establish the balance. Shower afterwards.

The apple cider vinegar helps the body become more alkaline. It also reduces the risks of arthritis. It will help with urinary tract infections and joint pain.

Figure 60 Apple cider vinegar soaks help the body move toward the alkaline pH range.

Maintain good elimination: Make certain your elimination pathways are open and working well. Food and toxins that sit around in your body start to decompose, and that decomposition results in an acid bodily environment. It's common knowledge among health professionals that people suffering from arthritis have been constipated for a long time, or had digestive problems that have negatively affected their elimination. Increasing your intake of whole food plant fiber through your diet and also through a whole food fiber supplement – can accomplish wonders.

Restore minerals: Most modern people are mineral deficient owing to poor soils on which food is grown. This leaves you with too few minerals with which your body can correct your pH. Therefore you might need to add mineral supplements. Alkalizing minerals are a major resource for reversing a pH that's too acidic. The primary alkalizing minerals are calcium, magnesium, sodium and potassium. Supplementing with these minerals may be a good choice while you work to change your diet and refill your body with the minerals that have become depleted over time.

If the above don't work, you may have some interference from unwanted visitors going on. Remember those parasites, bacteria, viruses and yeasts we talked about? They can make your pH run too acid and make it seem impossible to get it back in the normal range. So, if your pH correction efforts seem fruitless, this is a strong possibility. Work with your health practitioner to discover and eliminate these critters.

Restoring and maintain your pH balance in an overall neutral range can work wonders in addressing that troublesome joint pain, along with all those strange symptoms that are actually related after all.

***

Endnotes:

12-1. Each one-unit change in this scale corresponds to a ten-fold change in hydrogen ion concentration.
http://bio.groups.et.byu.net/pH_Biological_
fluids.phtml.

12-2. http://homeopathicremediesandtreatment.com/ Acid-base-Balance-Body-pH-Balance.php.

12-3. https://medlineplus.gov/ency/article/ 001183.htm.

12-4. https://www.healthline.com/health/acidosis# symptoms.

13. SPURS & CRYSTALS

"Everyone has inside them a piece of good news."
Anne Frank

I f you feel like you've got knives in your joints, or pieces of glass when you move, it's hard to imagine the possibility of being free to move without pain. Yet that's exactly the aim of working to dissolve arthritic spurs and crystals.

If you have spurs and crystals in your joints – those painful, solid pieces of matter, you don't have to be told they're a primary cause of arthritis. Their presence probably inspires a number of questions, perhaps, "Why would a body form stones? Or deposit what seems like sand into joints? And why would it make a bony spur – a sharp protrusion sticking out into the fluid space of a joint, where it pokes and causes such distress?"

Let's take a closer look at these conditions one at a time, starting with bony spurs, since they're so closely related to ph.

Bony spurs Bony spurs have much to do with acidity, a subject just addressed. You may recall that when your body is too acid, it can pull calcium, an alkalizing mineral, out of your bones and into your blood stream in a process it can carry out in less time than one heartbeat. That's part of its normal balancing process. However, delivering calcium from your bones to your blood requires a carrier, and that carrier is oils – omega 3 oils, specifically.

If you don't have enough omega 3 oils, your body can't complete that task. In this situation, your body starts to pull calcium out of your bones because it's needed for your blood, but doesn't have enough oils to complete the job. The result is an activity that's only partially completed, and the result is a bony spur in a joint.

Here's what this can look like if it occurs in your spine:

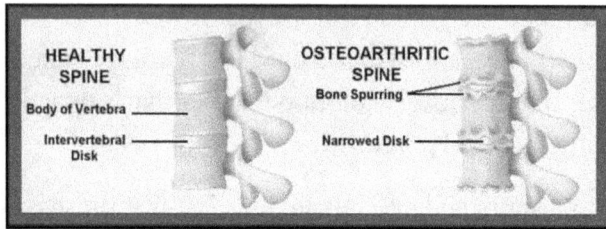

Figure 61 This is what bone spurs can look like in your spine.

A second reason bony spurs can form is not from lack of omega 3 oils, but from a disturbance in your oil metabolism. In other words, you might be consuming plenty of omega 3's, but there's a problem in your body's ability to break them down and render them bioavailable. In either case, the result can look like this:

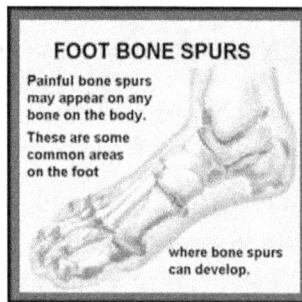

Figure 62 Here's where such bony spurs
can develop in your foot.

(When it comes to arthritis, the whole subject of oils is significant enough that we'll take it up in its own chapter, next.)

Crystal formation can also take place in your joints. There are two types of crystals that can form in your joints, each with a different composition. They can be differentiated medically when looking at fluid that's been aspirated from your joint and viewed under a microscope.

The first type, is called '*calcium pyrophosphate dihydrate*'. When you have these type of crystals in your joints, you may hear medical people refer to your condition as 'Pseudogout' or 'cppd disease'. They look like this:

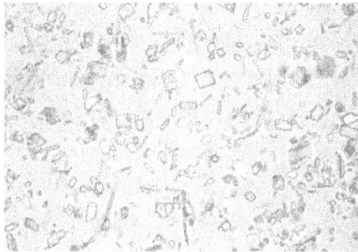

**Figure 63 Calcium pyrophosphate dihydrate crystals extracted
from synovial fluid, leading to a pseudogout diagnosis.**

The older you get, the more likely it is that any *acute* arthritis symptoms are caused by these crystals. You can suspect this with even greater confidence if your symptoms seem to have developed out of nowhere, and have started in your knee (although any joint can contain these crystals). You feel severe pain in the affected joint, and are likely to also see that it's red and swollen.

Although these symptoms might resolve on their own, they can also recur, even affecting several joints at once, most commonly in wrists, fingers and knees. (13-1)

This form of arthritis is a symptom of something out of whack with how you're breaking down food (your metabolism). If this is the case for you, you can also develop not only arthritic symptoms, but also gall stones, - even kidney stones. Happily, there are ways to proceed that can both explain your situation and give you a solution for it.

♋

WHAT YOU CAN DO

Reestablish Calcium/ Phosphorus Balance. The circumstance that can give rise to stone formation and crystals in joints is very common when your body's been fighting an infection or trying to get rid of a toxin. To do that, it has to make heat to burn it out. That's why you might have gotten a fever - your body was trying to burn that stuff up!

Regardless of *what* you've been trying to burn up, your body uses up a lot of phosphorus. (Phosphorus, as you may recall, is the substance on the end of a match that bursts into flame - i.e., makes heat - when given a bit of friction. It's also the substance that is used to ignite firecrackers.)

The longer your body has to make heat to rid itself of the substance(s), the more it uses your phosphorus stores, with the result that they get lower and lower, causing two problems. One, you lose more and more energy. That's because every energy molecule in your body has *three* phosphorus molecules on the end of it. (Its chemical name is ATP, or adeninetriphosphate). However, your body is starting to have too little phosphorus to continue to make the necessary energy molecules. That's why you get more and more fatigued, eventually able to just barely drag yourself around if it goes on long enough.

Second, you start forming these calcium crystals. Here's why: your body needs calcium to remain in liquid form so it can be used where it's needed. In solid form, your body can't use it. Keeping calcium in liquid form requires enough phosphorus in relation to calcium. In other words, with too little phosphorus, your calcium reverts to a solid form - crystals.

Now your body can't process it - can't use it and can't get rid of it. What are its choices then? If it can't get rid of it, the body's next option is that it tries to store it somewhere.

If it deposits those crystals in your gall bladder, they form gall stones, if in your kidney, kidney stones, if in the tympanic membrane in your ear, you can experience hearing loss. The membrane can't vibrate any more with those crystals in there. If they are deposited on your heart valve, the valve hardens and won't work right anymore, and if on the inside of your arteries, that causes hardening of the arteries.

What's the solution to bringing those calcium crystals back into solution? It's very straightforward: get your phosphorus levels back up high enough in relation to calcium so that the calcium comes back into solution! In an acute situation, health practitioners often recommend 30 drops of a liquid phosphorus supplement every ten minutes for two hours. This raises your phosphorus level, allowing the solidified calcium to come back into a liquid form, thus starting to dissolve the crystals. It also allows greater production of ATP – those wonderful energy molecules.

One other recommendation to prevent or reduce the possibility of stone formation: many people - especially women - take lots of calcium thinking it will protect their bones. However, often the products they're using are not balanced in relation to phosphorus. This, too, contributes to stone formation because of high calcium levels in relation to phosphorus. To avoid this, use a calcium that's balanced with phosphorus. The normal blood ratio is considered to be 4 parts of phosphorus to nine parts calcium. (13-2)

To stress the point – your body needs calcium and phosphorus to be in this proper ratio stated above. Therefore, it would be a bad move to decide to take a lot of phosphorus thinking you'd prevent these crystallizations and stones. Its best to work with a health practitioner who can evaluate your status and guide you so you can know when enough phosphorus is enough.

The second type of crystal is the one formed in actual gout, which is made of uric acid. Their long chemical name is 'monosodium urate monohydrate' crystals. Gout is one of the most painful forms of arthritis, usually developing in your big toe, but it can also occur in other joints. The symptoms are a result of sharp sensations of joint pain, like being poked with needles in the joint. And, of course, inflammation, redness, heat, swelling and joint stiffness develop too.

The crystals causing true gouty arthritis look like this under a microscope, where you can see how sharp they are:

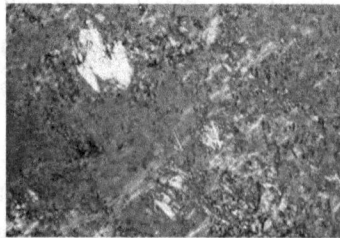

**Figure 64 Monosodium urate monohydrate crystals
taken from a gouty joint**

Medical treatment is based on removing the symptoms of pain and swelling. either with nonsteroidal anti-inflammatory drugs (nsaids, see Chapter 1)) or by removing fluid from the affected joint and injecting it with a glucocorticoid compound.

To address the underlying metabolic disturbance, one of the most commonly recommended strategies is to dramatically _decrease_ the amount of purines in your diet, because gouty crystals form from an excess of purines. Foods named below are those with high purine content, and therefore to be avoided:

Risk factors and symptoms to avoid

Gout commonly strikes between the ages of 30 and 50, usually occurring in men and, less often in women in menopause. Avoiding certain foods high in purine and keeping weight down are controllable risk factors.

Risky foods

Anchovies, herring/sardines

Mushrooms

Asparagus, peas and beans

Mussels

Kidney, liver, heart and brain, gravies, sweetbreads, broths and consomme

Alcohol increases production of urate acid and interferes with elimination

Other risk factors include sudden severe illness, crash diets, joint injury and chemotherapy

Joints affected

Urate crystals form in joints or cooler parts of the body

elbow

wrist

knee

ankle

Base of big toe

SOURCES: Arthritis Foundation, The Merck Manual of Medical Information   · AP

Figure 65 top foods to avoid due to their purine content if you have gout.

Health practitioners can also give you specific dietary recommendations based on your unique body. For example, digestive enzymes to help break down the proteins you're consuming, more hydrochloric acid to supplement your stomach acid, again to digest proteins more completely.

Increase the microcirculation in your kidneys with an herb such as Ginkgo biloba, an osmotic transfer supplement to help break down substances that were too large for your kidneys to filter.

Each recommendation will be based on your unique individual body. The point is, these and other things are actions you and your health practitioner can do so you don't have to continue suffering.

The bottom line is that bony spurs and crystal formations in your joints are basically solvable health challenges, not life sentences.

***

Endnotes:

13-1. http://www.arthritis.org/living-with-arthritis/tools-resources/expert-q-a/gout-questions/what-is-pseudogout.php.

13-2. http://www.betterhealthbytes.com/Volume-5-Issue-70.html.

14. NEED FOR LUBRICATION
A little progress every day adds up to big results.

Dry, creaky joints are not just painful, they also set the stage for joint inflammation and ultimately chronic arthritis. Happily, there are steps you can take both to prevent that unpleasant situation before it occurs, and to aid its reversal if already present.

To do so, you'll need to understand how your joints are lubricated. Luckily, it's quite simple, as there are only two main components: synovial fluid and articular cartilage.

Together they're a very slippery combination. They're:

"three times more slippery than skating on ice;
four to ten times more slippery than a metal-on-plastic hip replacement, and
more than thirty times as slippery as metal on metal using the best petroleum-based lubricant. " (14-1)

The images below represents the synovial fluid and articular cartilage. It illustrates the architecture of a healthy joint. The lubrication is carrying out its job effectively – minimizing both friction and wear. Imagine – or maybe you don't have to imagine it – putting pressure on some joint – perhaps stepping down onto a knee joint, without that effective lubrication!

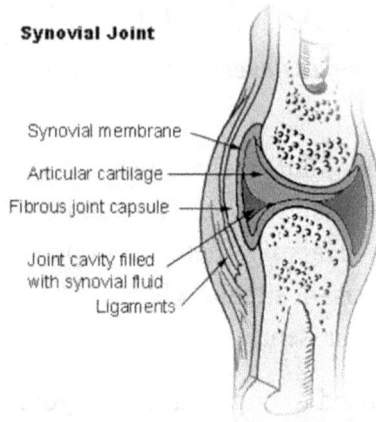

Synovial Joint

Synovial membrane

Articular cartilage

Fibrous joint capsule

Joint cavity filled
with synovial fluid

Ligaments

Figure 66 Notice the cavity of this joint - it contains synovial fluid, which helps protect the two bones from rubbing on each other, especially when they're put under pressure.

Here's an image to help you see what that's like:

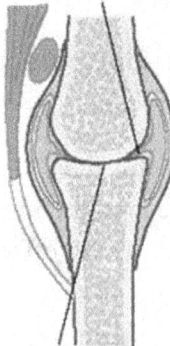

Eroded cartilage

**Bone ends
rub together**

Osteoarthritis

Figure 67 Compare the space between the two bones in the healthy joint image and this one, where effective lubrication is lacking.

ജ

WHAT YOU CAN DO

In the interest of preventing that uncomfortable condition, or addressing it if you already have it, requires two ingredients:

1. Consume the right oils (lipids) in sufficient quantity, and

2. Metabolize them effectively.

Why is this so important? Because the lubrication mechanisms in your joints - especially the synovial fluid - depends on a 'considerable amount of lipids." (14-2)

Needing these lipids, or oils is certainly not unique to arthritis suffers. You, along with everybody else, need the essential fatty acids (also referred to as EFA's or vitamin F). They are contained in this major food group of lipids, otherwise known as fats and oils.

Fats and oils are the building blocks your body uses to make everything from your brain cells (your brain is made up of 80% fat) to the insulation surrounding your nerves to your hormones to the walls of every cell in your body. It needs these EFA's in the form of sterols. To get sterols, it makes them from cholesterol which is made from dietary fat.

We've already covered some specifics in previous chapters about this food group that relate to arthritis. Here's a short review:

Use the right oils to control symptoms of arthritis pain Joint pain caused by inflammation can be relieved by an _oil_ component of food (gamma linolenic acid, covered in Chapter 2). This provides natural precursors your body needs to make its own anti-inflammatories. You will find the two greatest food concentrations in Black Currant Seed and Evening Primrose Oils.

Support your mineral bone-to-blood journey with oils. As detailed in Chapter 13, a carrier is required to deliver calcium from your bones to your blood, and that carrier is oils – omega 3 oils specifically. Without enough carrier oils you won't have enough calcium carriers. The result is partial completion of that bone-to-blood journey, and the result of that is a bony spur in your joint. Also, your body can't use this corrective device if your blood pH is too acid. (See Chapter 12 to review.)

Crystallizations and stones result from calcium absorption and delivery problems. Calcium is essential for muscle contraction, and that includes your heart muscle. When you don't have enough fatty acids present, (in the form of omega 3's) calcium lacks transportation to get delivered to where it's needed.

That's when your body will deposit calcium wherever it lands awaiting its transportation. This means it can land in your soft tissues, resulting in hardening of your arteries, deafness (if deposited in your tympanic membrane) or stone formation in your gall bladder or kidneys. (Again, Chapter 13 to review.)

Here's how you can you support this process to maintain the lubrication in your joints. The shortest answer, again, is that you will need to consume the *right kinds* of fats (or oils) from the lipid food group. These several types each have different uses and effects in your body. They're called by names that are probably familiar to you : unsaturated fats, saturated fats, trans fats and fake fats.

Are some fats better than others? Absolutely. When it comes to your arthritis, and also your health, some members of the family of essential fatty acids (EFA's) make excellent dinner guests, while others are best left uninvited. A closer look at each of these above categories will clarify which ones to include in your meal and which to avoid.

Include Enough Unsaturated Fats in Your Diet: The fatty acids you need to be sure to include are in the various polyunsaturated fats (or pufa's). Your body can't make these, but requires them for every living cell. The healthy family members of this lipid food group are linoleic acid (omega 6) and linolenic acid (omega 3).

Here's some of what the omega 6's in this essential dietary oils group do for you: (14-3)

- provide a high level of protection against cancer
- particularly of the breast
- contain lignans that get transformed by your intestinal bacteria
- are antibacterial
- are antifungal
- are antiviral
- stimulate skin and hair growth
- maintain bone health
- regulate your metabolism
- carry your fat soluble vitamins (A,D, E and K) from your gut to your tissues
- maintain your reproductive system
- support healthy growth, development and maintenance of your brain
- carry the various minerals your body needs to their destinations
- support your body's defenses against high cholesterol
- help defend against high blood pressure

- help decrease allergic responses
- help dissolve tumors
- help you attain and maintain a normal weight
- defend against heart disease, and
- defend against rheumatoid arthritis

Include Organic Olive Oil. Recent research has revealed that a compound found in olive oil (oleocanthal) prevents the production of inflammatory enzymes (cox-1 and cox-2) the same way the drug category of NSAIDS work (see Chapter 1). By comparison, 50 ml of olive oil, or about 3 1/2 tablespoons, is equal to a 200-mg tablet of ibuprofen. Since arthritis is basically an inflammatory response in your joints, you can grasp how important it is to provide your body with lots of these compounds because they both prevent and help resolve that inflammation. (14-4)

Food sources of omega-3s are found in these vegetable oils:

- flax seeds
- chia seeds
- wheat germ
- soybean oil
- walnuts
- pumpkin seeds
- canola oil
- red and black currant seeds
- fish oil.

Omega-6's are found in unsaturated vegetable oils such as

- soybean
- sunflower
- pumpkin

- primrose
- sesame
- grape seed
- borage
- legumes
- raw nuts
- seeds

Balance omega 3's and omega 6's. There's good reason not to go overboard with omega 6's. One reason is, those inflammatory enzymes (cox-2 enzymes) become more active and cause more joint inflammation in people who consume *large amounts* of omega-6 fatty acids.

If you're like most people consuming the typical Western diet, you get far too much omega-6 fat. That's because it's abundant in cooking oil, processed foods, fried foods, peanuts, and soy. Most guidelines suggest limiting omega-6 fat intake to no more than 3% to 5% of total calories. That can means reducing or eliminating fried foods and vegetable oil-laden fare.

Also, again, if you've been consuming a diet high in omega 6's, you'll need to pay extra attention to balancing your intake with an approximately *equal amount* of omega 3's.

Also, research has demonstrated that increasing omega-3 fats can help keep the inflammatory factors under control that cause cartilage destruction in arthritis. A study published in 2000 in the Journal of Biological Chemistry showed that omega-3 fatty acids offered a dose-dependent reduction in the expression of inflammatory cox-2 enzyme.

Most food sources contain a mix of both types of essential fatty acids. Olive oil is one such example, and it has demonstrated its usefulness in resolving inflammation. But, the one plant with the highest amount of efas, rich in omega 3, 6 and 9 is hemp. This plant is a cousin of the cannabis plant, but unlike marijuana, it contains none of the psychoactive ingredient, THC. Instead, it's more like hop or nettle, two other members of its family.

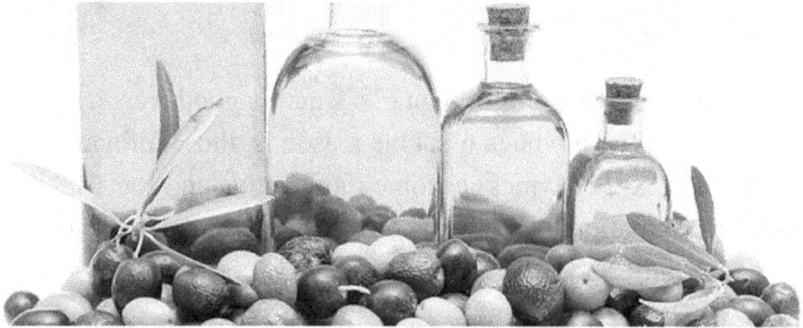

Figure 68 Including olive oil in your diet provides both omega 3s and omega 6s.

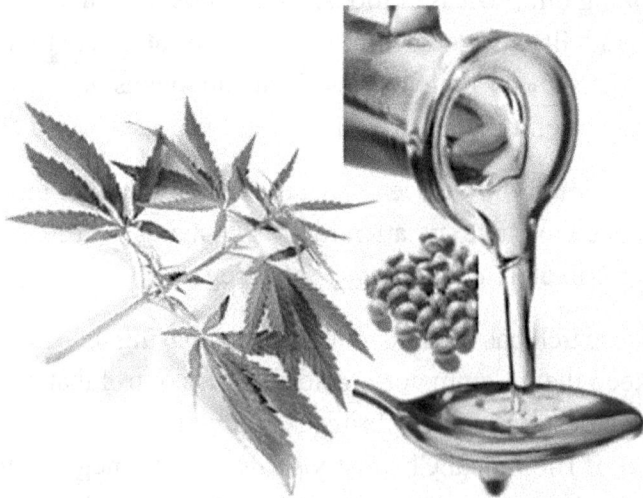

Figure 69 Add hemp seed oil to your diet to keep your joints well lubricated.

Consume saturated fats in moderation The relatives of unsaturated fats are saturated fats. They, too are also essential to your health. You may find this surprising, because they've been given a questionable reputation in the scientific community recently. This was due to the erroneous idea that they were a chief cause of coronary artery disease. This idea is falling away as awareness increases that inflammation is really what's at the root of coronary artery disease.

Saturated fats are found naturally in foods such as butter, cream, ghee, regular-fat milk and cheese, also in meats such as fatty cuts of beef, pork and lamb, including processed meats like salami, sausages and the skin on chicken and lard.

Eliminate transfatty acids Transfatty acids are found in margarine and any other product labeled "partially hydrogenated" or "hydrogenated". They're made in a laboratory by forcing hydrogen into polyunsaturated oil molecules under high temperature and pressure. They also form when vegetable oils are constantly reused, as in deep fried foods from fast food restaurants.

Evidence is mounting that links these transfatty acids to a variety of health problems, including heart disease and cancer. Consuming transfats, created by the mass commercial refinement of oils, strips your diet of the fatty acids that are so essential to your health and to the resolution of your arthritic symptoms. They also interfere with the formation of certain essential fatty acids (in particular, prostaglandins) that prevent tissue destruction and promote healing. In other words, transfats block the metabolic cascade the body uses to break down fats into the components your body can use for its various functions.

Transfats also confuse your body; they are sufficiently close to the good oils so your body uses them instead of the good fat. They should be outcasts from your diet because they are clearly toxic and dangerous. Finally, the FDA has agreed, determining that transfats (also called hydrogenated oils) are not generally recognized as safe, and set a three-year time limit for their removal from all processed foods. If this directive is carried out, that will eliminate them in the US in June, 2018.

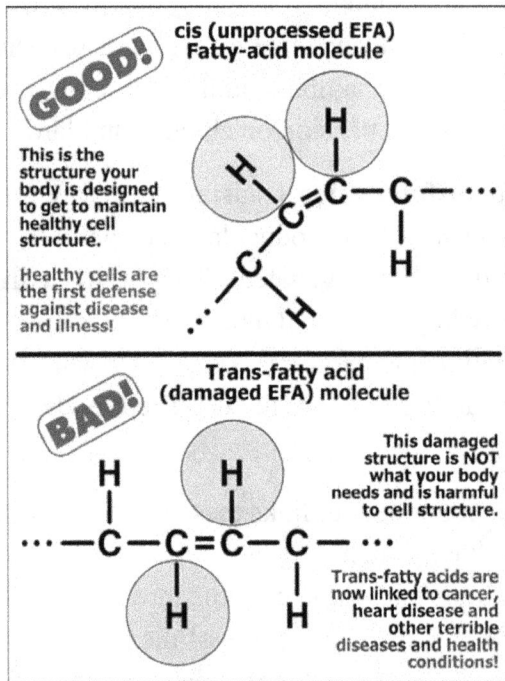

cis (unprocessed EFA) Fatty-acid molecule

GOOD!

This is the structure your body is designed to get to maintain healthy cell structure.

Healthy cells are the first defense against disease and illness!

Trans-fatty acid (damaged EFA) molecule

BAD!

This damaged structure is NOT what your body needs and is harmful to cell structure.

Trans-fatty acids are now linked to cancer, heart disease and other terrible diseases and health conditions!

Figure 70 Be sure to read labels on foods before purchase to make sure you're not buying harmful transfats.

Avoid fake fats. New arrivals on the food choice scene are the category of fats called fake fats. They have a variety of brand names. For example, one is called Olean, with the trademark name of olestra. According to the center for science in the public interest (cspi), Olean has been shown to cause diarrhea, loose stools, intestinal cramping and other gastrointestinal symptoms including fecal incontinence. Some people have even been hospitalized as a result of these symptoms.

Be sure to read labels on foods before purchase to make sure you're not buying harmful transfats.

Some companies are now manufacturing epoprostenol, or prostacyclin. These fake fats are synthetically produced to attempt to "reverse vascular lesions". Fake fats rob your body of nutrients, in part by interfering with the absorption of carotenoids, a family of fat soluble nutrients that have been associated with lowering the risk of cardiovascular disease and cancer. Nonetheless, the Food and Drug Administration has approved their use. However, these vascular lesions can also be reversed by balancing the EFA (or ecosanoid) system by proper eating.

Before leaving this subject, let's return to the two main mechanisms your joints use to stay flexible: synovial fluid and articular cartilage. Remember that the two together make a exceptionally slippery combination. Much of that is due to the fact that the synovial membrane secretes – almost oozing – a continuous supply of hyaluronic acid. This is key to generating that slippery, viscous, lubricating fluid, almost like gelatin, that's called the synovial fluid. That's why it's often offered as a supplement to assist dry, creaky joints.

While this sounds great, the fact is that hyaluronic acid only exists for an extremely short time before your body breaks it down. Indeed, there's scant scientific evidence that taking an HA supplement does any good. Animal studies demonstrated that only a small amount was even absorbed after taking it orally. For that reason, the best strategy is to support its production rather than supplementing it from some external source. An approach for doing so is summarized below.

To summarize:

Keep yourself well hydrated. Remember that the lubricating agent in your joints is first of all a liquid. Don't allow yourself to get dehydrated, especially when working out and causing greater stress on your joints. Drink plenty of good, clean, clear water – at least 8 ounces 8 times a day, and more if exercising or sweating.

Balance your fat intake to keep yourself "well-oiled". Over the period of a month, your body needs about equal parts of omega 3's, omega 6's and omega 9's (your body can make this last type). Balancing your fat intake in this way allows each type to work in concert with the others. Plus, you avoid an imbalance, which could otherwise shut down your entire system. In addition, because exposure in modern life to chemicals and radiation depletes your body of essential fatty acids (efa's, or vitamin F), you'll need to pay attention to actively resupplying them anyway.

This right balance of EFAs, adds emminent alternative health author Ann Louise Gittleman, M.S., "will allow you to lose weight effortlessly and painlessly without becoming preoccupied with dieting. Essential fat is the healthiest and easiest way to attain and maintain your normal weight." (14-5)

Make sure you digest your oils well. A note about oils: to benefit from your intake, you will need to digest them well, and that requires good bile flow in your liver. If you have light colored stools, you can bet you've got a bile flow problem, so check with your health practitioner to develop a strategy to correct it.

Maintain high levels of hyaluronic acid. To start this means consuming foods that contain especially high levels, such as potatoes and other root vegetables like carrots and sweet potatoes. Also consume leafy green vegetables such as kale and spinach. You will also find high concentrations of hyaluronic acid in Asian vegetables such as imoji, konyaku and satoimo. Hyaluronic acid is sensitive to heat and cooking destroys it. To avoid this problem, eat many of the sources raw, such as carrots and spinach leaves, perhaps in salads or snacks. (14-6)

Also, include plenty of nutrients your body uses to both make hyaluronic acid and to break it down, giving room for a fresh supply. Minerals needed for this activity include magnesium, zinc, and sulfur to create it, along with iron and vitamin C for removing old HA molecules.

Magnesium You'll find magnesium in almonds, bananas, chocolate, legumes, pumpkin seeds, spinach and Swiss chard.

Zinc Good sources for zinc are in chickpeas, dark chocolate, cashews, almonds, yogurt, and pumpkin seeds.

Sulfur sources include garlic and cruciferous vegetables (broccoli, cabbage, cauliflower kale and turnips.

Iron Dark green, leafy vegetables are rich in iron, as are raisins. Last, vitamin C is plentiful in citrus fruits, strawberries, kiwi fruit, pineapple, cantaloupe, tomatoes, sweet bell peppers, and parsley.

Avoid low fat diet; Every cell and function of your body requires fats to function and stay healthy.

In short, both scientific research and practical experience demonstrates providing your body with the types of fats it needs does, in fact, have an impact on the potential development of arthritis and its degree of severity if present. To avoid arthritis entirely, and to minimize its progression if it's started, keep yourself well oiled!

***

Endnotes

14-1. https://www.slideshare.net/debasismukherjee20/joint-lubrication-by-dr-debasis-mukherjee.

14-2. http://www.mdpi.com/2075-4442/1/4/102/htm.

14-3. https://www.drweil.com/vitamins-supplements-herbs/vitamins/balancing-omega-3-and-omega-6/

14-4. http://www.todaysdietitian.com/newarchives/040212p12.shtml.

14-5. Excerpted from the article *"Dietary Fats and Their Food Sources"* Pamela Levin R.N. published by the Nourishing Company, 2005.

14-6. https://www.livestrong.com/article/38313-retain-hyaluronic-acid-body/

15. MECHANICAL STRESS & INJURIES
"It's not stress that kills us, it is our reaction to it."

– Hans Selye

Perhaps you were steaming away on a computer project, or you were hammering away with hammer and nails, or kicking a soccer ball down the field. And then there was that telltale signal you'd gone too far – a sharp pain, or a dull spreading one, and you know you've injured a joint.

You have that slow, dawning fear, that life as you know it is over. You can't complete the project or the game – you are sidelined. While that may be true in the short term, joint injuries due to mechanical stress and injuries *do not have to be life sentences.*

To find out what you can do to make certain they're not, check out the following definitions and guidelines. And be reassured – all is not lost!

When any of your joints break down because it's overstressed or overused, it's suffered a 'mechanical stress injury', or a 'repetitive stress injury'. Any joint in your body can be affected, - your little finger, your knee, shoulder, back or any other place where two bones meet.

After any joint is physically injured, it can develop a type of arthritis is called post- traumatic arthritis. In the U.S., post-traumatic arthritis accounts for about 12% of osteoarthritis of the hip, knee, and ankle, which means that about 5.6 million people are affected.

Overstresses or overuse set the stage for arthritis because the joint is no longer cushioned properly, while physical injury sets the stage because the joint has been damaged in some way. Together, such joint injuries account for a 20-fold or more increase in the risk of developing osteoarthritis. (15-1)

These are best prevented, so we'll cover that subject first, and then deal with what to do if you have such an injury.

❧

WHAT YOU CAN DO

Prevention: Pay attention to how you use a computer keyboard. Since the most common cause of mechanical stress induced arthritis in this modern age is computer keyboard use. No doubt either you or someone you know has been diagnosed with carpal tunnel syndrome. It's a repetitive stress injury to the wrist that's becoming more and more common as people spend many hours typing on keyboards. Keep your wrist relatively straight and don't subject it to sharp, bent angles. However, that won't in and of itself be sufficient.

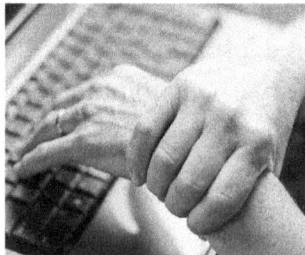

Figure 71 Carpal tunnel syndrome is so common now due to lengthy or repeated use of a keyboard.

Prevention: Proper Spinal Alignment. Spinal misalignment sets the stage for arthritis. You might think of your spine or sacroiliac joints when you think of bones out of their proper relationship to each other, but actually any place where two bones meet can become misaligned. Sometimes, these joints have been misaligned before birth, and sometimes a disease process such as a bone fracture or even bone cancer can be at the root of a joint wearing down more quickly than normal.

Prevention: Keep good alignment when sitting, especially at a keyboard. That's the major way to prevent mechanical stress injury from long hours at a computer. So significant is this factor in creating arthritis, that the country of Malaysia went to a great deal of effort to design optimal work areas specifically formulated to create good body mechanics. These were based on the average measurements of the Malaysian body while sitting at a computer: (15-2)

Department of Mechanical and Materials Engineering
Faculty of Engineering and Built Environment
Universiti Kebangsaan Malaysia

MALAYSIAN ANTHROPOMETRICS DATA			
Data No. :		Age :	
State origin :		Date of birth :	
Sex :		Religion :	
Race :		Occupation :	

ANTHROPOMETRY DATA	UNIT/mm	ANTHROPOMETRY DATA	UNIT/mm
1. Stature		7. Popliteal height	
2. Shoulder breadth		8. Sitting knee height	
3. Chest depth		9. Forearm hand length	
4. Sitting height		10. Sitting elbow height	
5. Sitting eye height		11. Thigh clearance	
6. Sitting shoulder height		12. Head length	

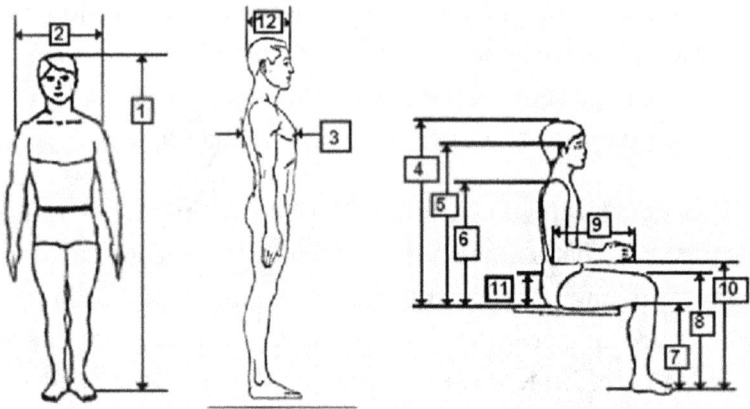

Figure 72 The unique proportions of Malaysians were averaged to design an arthritis-preventing work station.

Although your bodily measurements may be different from 90% of Malaysians, you can still use the two sections of the above chart to create your own optimally designed computer station.

Prevention: Good Body Mechanics. Use good body mechanics when carrying out any task. We've already addressed how to do that when using a computer. Three basic pointers can assist you in other situations:

1. When standing, do so with your feet apart to create a sturdy foundation.
2. When bending, bend at your knees instead of your waist.
3. When moving, keep your neck, back, hips, and feet aligned; avoid twisting and bending at the waist.

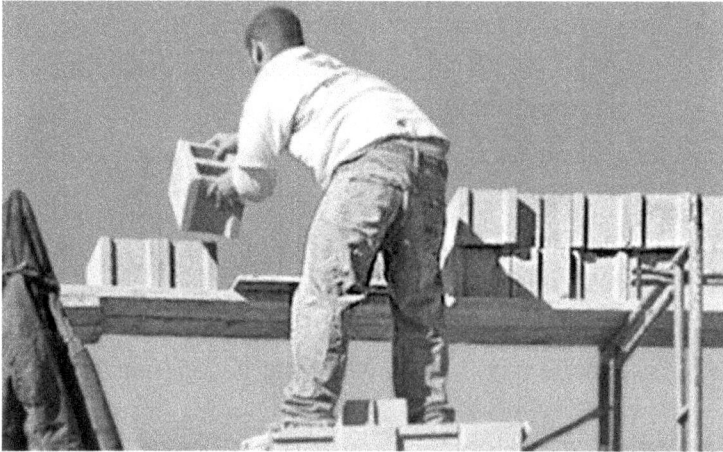

Figure 73 This worker needs strong ligaments and muscles to help prevent a repetitive stress injury of his back, knees and wrists. He also needs good body mechanics, which means bending at his knees instead of his waist.

If carrying out a particular repetitive movement at work or during sports, take moments to pause, stretch the area and move it through its normal range of motion. This increases circulation, flushes out any toxins and stretches any areas that were pinched.

Prevention: Strengthen muscles and ligaments, especially if you have a mechanical stress injury in your back. Excessive use in work or sports is huge arthritis-inducing category which can lead to strains, falls, ruptured discs. These are a result of high stress and even breaks, any of which can lead to the necessity for surgery.

Prevention: Keep core muscles strong. Keeping your core muscles and their ligaments strong and in good working order is a top way to minimize the likelihood you'll develop arthritic problems in your back. If your abdominal muscles are weak and the muscles of the back are weak in general, you'll put more stress on the joints in your back and cause arthritic pain and symptoms.

- in your arm to protect your elbow if your occupation involves digging, mining, using compressed air power tools or mining
- in your arms and shoulders to protect your elbows, wrists and shoulders if you use a pneumatic drill.
- in your lower and upper legs and core abdominal muscles if you typically carry heavy loads
- in your hands to protect your fingers if you do small repetitive movements with your hands (needlework, dressmaking, piano-playing, diamond-cutting). (15-3)

Since playing certain sports can also create joint loading that sets up arthritis, be sure to condition yourself accordingly:

- if you play rugby, strengthen your neck to avoid cervical spondylosis
- if you play tennis, strengthen you upper and lower arms to avoid tennis elbow
- if you ski, strengthen your upper and lower thighs to protect your knees.

Prevention: Change the way you use a joint whenever possible. It's often the repetitive use of a joint that sets up arthritis. That means you can greatly reduce the chances you'll develop it if you vary how you use it and how often you use it. As the Cleveland Clinic, which specializes in such injuries points out, "such injuries can damage the cartilage and/or the bone, changing the mechanics of the joint and making it wear out more quickly. The wearing-out process is accelerated by continued injury and excess body weight."(15-4)

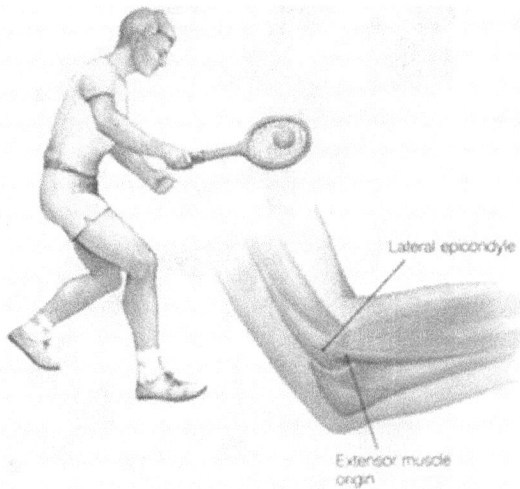

Figure 74 'Tennis elbow' is a mechanical stress injury

Prevention: Don't overdo workouts. Intense cardio workouts can be especially hard on joints. This is particularly true for women - the combination of the female anatomy along with such highly demanding activity causes spiking of adrenaline and cortisol. When cortisol is high, the normally joint protective ligaments become looser at a time there is high physical load on joints. (15-5)

If you use a wheelchair user, take care not to jerk your shoulders when manually propelling the chair.

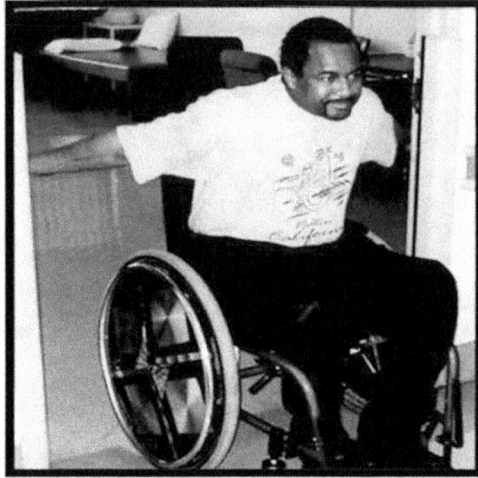

Figure 75 This man's shoulders are vulnerable.

Prevention: Maintain normal weight. is a condition that overloads joints, tearing them down and causing pain. Your joints are designed to take only so much weight, but they have to cushion a great deal more impact when you're overweight. For example, let's say your normal weight is 150 pounds. Since your knees carry about 1 ½ times your body weight when you walk on a level surface, if you weigh 200-pounds instead, your knees carry 300 pounds of pressure with each step.

On an incline, the pressure on each knee increases to two to three times your body weight, or 400-600 pounds. When you squat to tie a shoelace or pick up an item you dropped, the load on each knee goes up to go up to four or five times your body weight, or 600-1000 pounds!

But, that's only part of how extra weight can set the stage for arthritis. When you carry too much weight for your frame, your body will produce certain inflammatory factors that can contribute to trouble in your other joints (for example, in your hands). (15-6)

Keep your weight as close to your ideal as possible. Decide: do you need to lose weight? The current most commonly accepted way to answer that question is to determine your body mass index. In general, a body mass index of 25 to 29.5 is considered 'overweight', while one of 30 or more is considered 'obese'.

In terms of your overall health and longevity, recent research reveals that it may not be the amount of fat you carry. Rather where you carry it and whether or not it is accompanied by inflammation seem to be the primary threats to your overall health. What this means is that if your fat is stored in fat cells and not in your organs (your liver, pancreas, heart, etc), you have no diabetes, your insulin is low and you have no excess blood fat, you're likely to stay pretty healthy.

However, there's still the possibility of developing arthritis to consider. The weight-carrying stress on your joints is still taking place, so it's best to keep your weight under control and as close to your ideal weight range as possible.

Weight loss can be a frustrating process, yet losing a few pounds can go a long way toward reducing the pressure on your knees — and protecting them. For example, research has proven that a sustained 10- to 15-pound weight loss in obese young people can translate to a much lower risk of osteoarthritis later in life." (15-7)

HOW TO KNOW IF YOU'VE OVERDONE IT.
You'll experience symptoms similar to other types of arthritis: joint pain, swelling, fluid accumulation in the joint and decreased tolerance for walking, sports, stairs, and other activities that stress the joint.

Post-traumatic arthritis can result in the development of scar tissue in and/or around the joint. To soften it, and thus allow the joint to function more easily, you might consider castor oil packs, wheat germ oil, sesame seed oil and certain homeopathic remedies designed for that purpose.

Resolving scar tissue in that way has an added bonus: because parasites, bacteria and viruses love to live in scar tissue, it eliminates these tissues where these invaders can take up residence.

HOW TO AID HEALING FOR MECHANICAL AND POST-TRAUMATIC STRESS INJURIES

Happily, with good body mechanics and correction of the injury, you can eliminate most joint stresses and thus prevent arthritis altogether or reverse it if it's begun. And if you have a post-traumatic stress injury, there is also a great deal you can do to promote healing and tissue repair. Here are some pointers for doing so:

Use the stages of healing below. If you've started to develop a problem in your joints, whether from mechanical injury or post-trauma, use the following stages of healing to determine what you need to do and when you need to do it. That will maximize the possibility of reversing it.

Phases of tissue healing

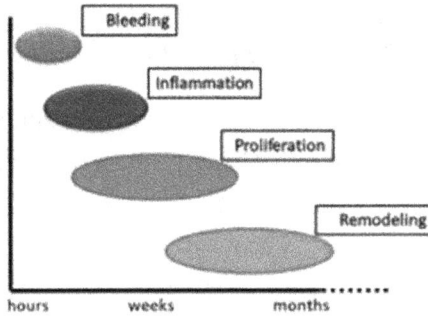

Figure 76 Each phase of healing has its own optimum requirements for rest, nutrition and exercise.

Initial Stage: Address it immediately. This first chart illustrates how important it is to deal with any injury in its earliest stage – the first 48 hours. That's because this is the crucial time period immediately following the injury where cell function is declining but is still reversible.

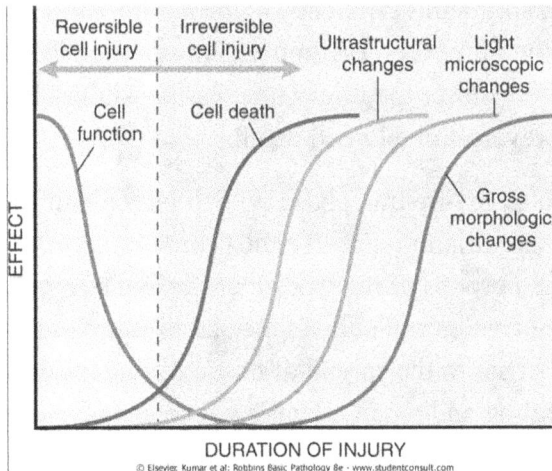

Figure 77 Early intervention may prevent cell death and irreversible changes.

Initial Stage: Address shock. If you're in shock from an acute injury, you'll need to come out of shock to start the healing process. In addition to the medical care you receive, you can use Rescue Remedy (a Bach flower remedy).

Then, in the immediate moments following a mechanical stress injury, the standard protocol for attending to it is represented by the acronym R.I.C.E., which means: (15-8).

> **R**est
> **I**ce
> **C**ompression and
> **E**levation.

Initial Stage: Rest. There is absolutely no substitute for rest – no supplement, no magic pill. If the joint was overused or suffered an acute trauma, it needs rest. That means not just in the immediate moments following the injury, but also during the days following. This allows the healing process to take place at maximum speed and efficiency. During this early post-trauma period is the time when the injury is most reversible. The longer the time frame after the injury, the less possibility there is of complete reversal due to cell death.

In this acute post-trauma phase (which lasts about 48 hours), bleeding and inflammation are the primary processes taking place. The purpose of this bodily pre-response is to deliver effector molecules and cells to the site of injury, to form a physical barrier to the spread of tissue damage and to initiate wound healing and repair. That's why rest, ice, compression and elevation are so effective here, as they help control and manage that response. Compression bandages or garments designed for the area (ankle, wrist, knee, etc) can provide major assistance.

Apply ice directly to the injured area for no more than 15 minutes followed by at least 15 minutes off and then repeat the process. This creates blood vessel constriction followed by constriction fatigue that results in a deep relaxation.

Initial Stage: Good Nutrition. Of course, good general nutrition is essential - particularly plenty of protein. Whatever amount of protein you had been consuming, you can estimate that you will need about 30 grams extra for your healing and repair process. You'll also need foods rich in enzymes – which means those that are raw.

Initial Stage: These Herbs are Helpful. Herbs can be of major assistance in controlling pain and supporting healing. The following are excellent for managing initial inflammation and continuing throughout the healing process.

- Boswellia,
- Turmeric,
- Celery Seed fruit and
- Ginger rhizome

Initial Stage: Arnica Montana. As the affected area becomes increasingly red, swollen, painful and hot, the compounds in Arnica can modulate this inflammatory response, assist in dissipating old blood and fluids confined in the area, and decrease bruising. Arnica aids wound healing.

Initial Stage: Avoid vasodilators. However, don't take the oils of Black Currant Seed or Evening Primrose during this first phase because they cause vasodilation, which means they contribute to bleeding in traumatized blood vessels. They will be helpful later.

Initial Stage: Include Sesame Oil. However, you can use Sesame oil, which supports products of thrombocytes, as it's not only proven useful, but beneficial. Extra zinc is also excellent to promote the healing process.

Initial Stage: Traumeel. A product from Germany called *Traumeel* is an excellent supportive product for the acute stage of traumatic injury for dealing with pain and inflammation. It's available in tablets, drops, injection solution, ointment, and gel.

Initial Stage: Lightest Possible Touch Only. Avoid massage directly on the site of injury at this time except the lightest possible touch. Massage above and below the injury is fine.

MIDDLE PHASE HEALING AND REPAIR

In the middle phase, which begins about 48 hours after the injury and can last up to six weeks, your body moves out of its acute response and into an inflammatory and proliferatory phase. This is where the major tissue healing process takes place. Here, you can assist the vessels that carry new cells in and remove old, damaged ones by creating 'vascular gymnastics.' You rotate using a hot water bottle on the affected area for 5-6 minutes followed by an ice pack for 2-3 minutes and repeat that three times total.

Use These Oils to Manage Inflammation This is the time to add plenty of Black Currant Seed Oil or Evening Primrose Oil to provide the precursors your body uses to make anti-inflammatories.

These Herbs and Supplements are Helpful Now To support tissue and capillary healing and integrity here, consider adding the herb Gotu Kola, along with a product rich in bioflavonoids, such as one containing rutin, hesperiden, Quercetin. A whole food vitamin C product also supports tissue repair and healing. To support your veins, consider the herb Horse Chestnut. Continue enzyme-rich foods and a high protein intake.

Support Circulatory Repair, Nerve Conduction and Good Blood Supply If circulation has been compromised, consider Ginkgo Biloba, which promotes microcirculation.

Good nerve conduction is essential for the muscles around a joint to function well and protect it, while a good blood supply is required to carry the oxygen and nutrients that feed the joint, remove carbon dioxide and eliminate waste.

If nerves have been compromised, the following can support repair:

- a blend of Skullcap
- St. John's Wort
- Schizandra
- Saffron stigma
- Inositol (a B vitamin)
- Omega 3 fatty acids (such as that in flaxseed oil).

LAST, REMODELING, HEALING AND REPAIR PHASE

The healing work of the last stage involves removing the inflammatory elements from the tissue so that it can return to normal structure or function. The increased vascular permeability of the previous two stages is reversed, all inflammatory byproducts and dead cells are removed and tissue cells are regenerated.

The above herbs and nutrients in the middle stages of healing can be continued into this last or remodeling phase.

Last, Remodeling Healing and Repair Phase. Deep Heat, Vigorous Massage and Exercise. If your injury has reached this chronic stage, you can use deep heat for up to 15 minutes at a time. The work of this stage also benefits greatly from exercise. Bicycling and swimming are both exercises that are fairly easy on joints, but talk with your health professional to get routines that are specific for your best healing. This last stage is also the time to introduce more vigorous massage.

Deal with Scar Tissue If this work is not possible to complete in this third stage for whatever reason, your body will generate fibrous tissue (scar tissue.) .

If scar tissue has been generated, your health practitioner can assist you with procedures and remedies to help resolve it. This might consist of one or more of the following:

- using castor oil packs (instructions for how to carry this out are available online),
- taking Sesame Seed Oil or Wheat Germ Oil internally plus locally over the scarred area
- using homeopathic remedies formulated to resolve scar tissue

The take-away message is, that no matter what stage your mechanical stress injury is in currently – whether hours old or years old – there are measures you can take to address it and bring about the healing that will restore better functioning.

***

Endnotes:

15-1. https://www.ncbi.nlm.nih.gov/pmc/articles/
PMC4109888/#bibr9-1947603513495889.

15-2. https://www.researchgate.net/publication/
283159577_Recommended_Chair_and_Work_Surfaces_Dimens
ions_of_VDT_Tasks_for_Malaysian_
Citizens.

15-3. http://www.arthrolink.com/en/osteoarthritis-folders/all-
folders/osteoarthritis-and-work.

15-4. https://my.clevelandclinic.org/health/diseases/
14616-post-traumatic-arthritis.

15-5. https://www.mindbodygreen.com/articles/is-your-workout-
messing-with-your-hormones.

15-6. https://www.health.harvard.edu/pain/why-weight-matters-
when-it-comes-to-joint-pain.

15-7. Ibid.

15-8. https://www.mayoclinic.org/first-aid/first-aid-
sprain/basics/art-20056622.

16. AUTOIMMUNE REACTION

You have been assigned this mountain
to show it can be moved.

If you're diagnosed with an arthritic autoimmune disease (autoimmune arthritis), you can feel pretty hopeless. You might even start to distrust your body – or at least your immune system – thinking it has turned against you.

If you're told you have rheumatoid arthritis, you'll likely know that's considered to be autoimmune in origin, meaning that your immune system is attacking your own joints.

Now, in addition to that painful condition, you might even assume that searching for answers is fruitless and that you are simply doomed to live with these painful, swollen joints.

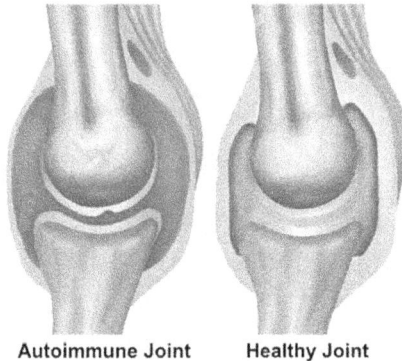

Autoimmune Joint   Healthy Joint

Figure 78 One of the key differences between a joint being attacked by its own immune system and a healthy joint is massive inflammatory response.

However, all is not lost. There is a growing consensus among health practitioners and scientists that any autoimmune problem – including autoimmune arthritis, or rheumatoid arthritis – is the result of a *confused* or *dysfunctional* immune system. Further, they conclude that the reason(s) for this chaotic situation can be identified and eliminated, so your immune system can return to its normal working order.

That viewpoint means you can take constructive action in sleuthing out what's confusing your immune system. You can address what you discover to resolve your condition. All of a sudden, you're no longer doomed! So, let's get to what can create this dysfunction or dysregulation or confusion.

A massive inflammatory response is one key difference between a healthy joint and one attacked by its own immune system. To be clear, autoimmunity is an attack on a target organ that your immune system no longer recognizes as self, attacking your joints instead. (16-1) The result looks like this:

RHEUMATOID ARTHRITIS

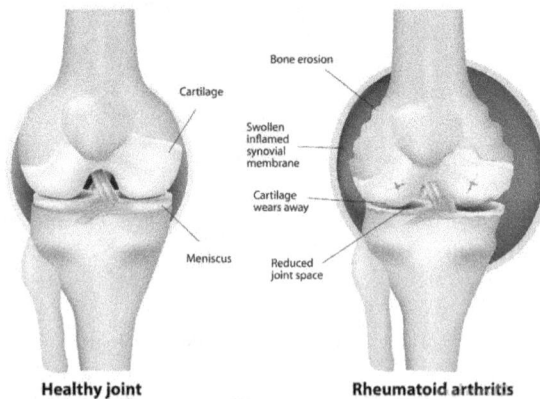

Healthy joint   Rheumatoid arthritis

Figure 79 Your own immune system can cause the inflammation, bone erosion and cartilage damage seen in this joint on the right.

What are some possible factors that can contributors to your immune system becoming confused or dysfunctional? The short (and possibly shocking!) Answer is, that any of the subjects we've covered previously can create the immune confusion that leads to autoimmune arthritis!

What's happening at a physical level is that your immune cells – the T cells (or various thrombocytes) that respond like an army of soldiers to create that initial inflammation in your joints have now gotten confused. They're failing to recognize the difference between substances and tissues your body makes normally and those that are foreign. They're making a big mistake - attacking your own tissues. In the case of autoimmune arthritis, they're attacking your joints.

୨

WHAT YOU CAN DO

To take a closer look at some factors that can contribute to this confusion, let's start by returning to the subject of foods (first addressed in Chapter 3). How could they be a potential cause of confusing your immune system? After all, you might think, since you consume them to nourish your body, they couldn't be the source of your arthritis. However, that would be entirely incorrect.

Learn Your Food Intolerances and Avoid Consuming Them. To discover how the foods you eat can underlie and diagnosis of autoimmune arthritis, consider a component of food called 'lectins'. Lectins are large protein molecules in food. They can bind with carbohydrates which then can bind to cell membranes in your joints. In other words, lectins create a way for their food molecules to stick together with your own cells in your joints while bypassing your own immune system.

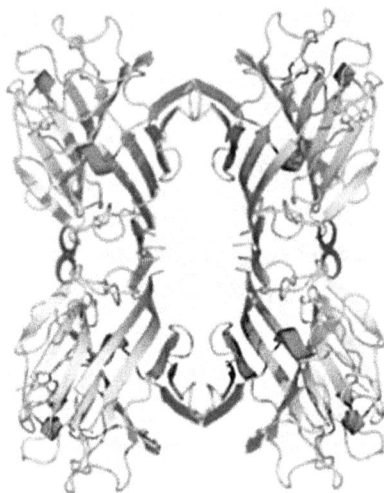

Figure 80 This Lectin is Leucoagglutinin, a toxic phytohemagglutinin found in raw Vicia faba (fava beans).

Lectins can cause havoc in your joints three ways. One, they can increase inflammation (by stimulating ifn-gamma, il-1, and tnf-alpha production). Two, they can bind to a particular molecule (sialic acid) in the synovial fluid in joints. And third, since lectins can act as triggers for your immune system, they can cause autoimmunity in susceptible people. (16-2)

Does this mean you need to avoid foods that are high in lectins? The answer to that is, perhaps, but not necessarily. That's because you may not be susceptible to the lectins in that particular food, but may be susceptible to those in some other food or food group.

For example, high lectin foods include beans, cereal grains, seeds, nuts, and potatoes. Some of these may be harmful to you if you eat a great deal of them, or perhaps only if you consume them in an uncooked or improperly-cooked form. Some people are highly sensitive to lectins in nightshades (potatoes, tomatoes, peppers, tobacco, eggplant) and others are not. So when it comes to foods, the task is to discover if there are foods that are confusing _your_ immune system, rather than what foods are high in lectins.

You may have noticed the phrase 'in susceptible people' in the above description. That raises the questions:, "Am I a susceptible person?" and if so, "What can I do about it?" To find answers, some people have benefitted by following recommendations for their blood type as identified by Peter D'Adamo in his book _Eat Right for Your Type_. (16-3) Also, getting tested by a health professional competent to discover your unique food vulnerabilities will prove especially valuable. (If you need to find such a practitioner, see Chapter 18.)

Meanwhile, keep in mind that being susceptible to particular lectins is _not the same as having an allergic response to them_. Many people have gone to an allergist, undergone expensive and uncomfortable allergy scratch tests, (as outlined in Chapter 3) changed their diets radically and had no appreciable change in their arthritic symptoms.

To understand why, remember the way lectins work. To repeat: lectins create a way for their food molecules to stick together with your own cells in your joints _while bypassing your own immune system._ In short, lectins can confuse your immune system's ability to determine what's you and what's not you, but not cause an allergic response in so doing.

Consume Foods Rich in Polyphenols. While you may need to avoid lectins in certain foods, there are also foods to eat as much as possible. These are foods rich in polyphenols – particular antioxidants that reduce inflammation and slow cartilage destruction. Green tea is packed with them along with another antioxidant (epigallocatechin-3-gallate (egcg)) that blocks the production of the molecules that cause joint damage in rheumatoid arthritis. Other foods rich in polyphenols include dark chocolate, pomegranates, blueberries and other dark berries.

Eliminate Infectious Agents. As pointed out earlier, any of the subjects of the previous chapters, or any combination of them, can dysregulate your immune system, causing it to become confused about what's you and what's not you, making the mistake that mounts an attack on the wrong cells – namely those in your joints.

Let's take a closer look at one other major category –all the various immune challenges we've discussed previously: Lyme and Lyme vectors, parasites, viruses, bacterial infections, yeast, fungus, mold and candida.

Each of these has its own ways of disrupting and confusing your immune system – after all, that's how they manage to survive and thrive in your body. Bacteria not only steal your resources; they can emit toxins your immune system finds perplexing (me or not me? not sure…) Bacteria adjust themselves to survive antibiotics; MRSA, or Methicillin-resistant staph aureus is just one such example. Hospital environments are loaded with such bugs that are antibiotic resistant.

Viruses, too, can cover themselves with protein coats that are the same or closely resemble those of normal cells in your joints, fooling your immune system into thinking 'this is me'. Viruses literally get inside your cells, hijack your DNA and start bossing it around, telling it what to do. Your immune system no doubt sees the cell containing the virus as 'me' –after all, it's a normal cell , but then there's something decidedly 'not me' about it. Shall it get attacked and eliminated or not?

Parasites have learned over millennia not just to coexist, but also co-evolve with human beings. They've also learned to modulate and evade human immune defenses. (16-4) Some emit substances that cloud their presence, some coat their eggs in human-looking proteins, some even use your joints as their nursery, laying their eggs to gestate in that protected environment and so forth.

Meanwhile, Candida and many of these other living entities actually hang on to toxic metals. Apparently they find this helps them evade immune attacks because heavy metals are immunosuppressive.

The solution to any of these situations is to eliminate the bugs as we've covered in greater detail in previous chapters.

Non-prescription choices. Happily, rounds and rounds of antibiotics -with their microbiome-eradicating aftermath - are not your only choice. To remind you, there are:

Whole food products concentrated to clinical potency (available through many licensed health practitioners). These support your bodily processes and provide the substances any particular organ or system needs to rebuild;

Whole organic herbs These support your immune system while providing substances these immune challenges find incompatible with residence in your body, and

Homeopathic remedies These 'remind' your body about how to respond effectively to these unwanted invaders.

Your health practitioner can best advise you which particular ones to choose.

Rehmannia glutinosa root especially helps to deconfuse autoimmune conditions.

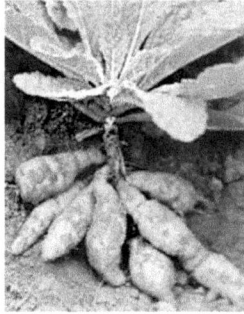

Figure 81 Rehmannia root helps deconfuse the immune system.

Chinese herbalists have used it hundreds of years for various benefits - as multi-purpose tonic, to build up kidney function and urinary tract health (especially in men), to upgrade the cardiovascular system and normalize cholesterol levels, blood circulation, digestion, deafness, vertigo and sexual health and as a tonic for anti-aging.

However, its therapeutic effect for deconfusing the immune system is what makes it so often recommended for autoimmune conditions. Although the mechanisms by which it helps this process are unclear, still it's considered by many health practitioners to be a standard herbal recommendation for any autoimmune condition.

Armed with this knowledge, you can see that a diagnosis of 'autoimmune arthritis' can serve as a direction for where to discover your healing, rather than a condition you are required to endure.

Endnotes:

16-1. https://www.ncbi.nlm.nih.gov/pmc/articles/pmc1618732/ .

16-2. https://en.wikipedia.org/wiki/.

16-3. http://www.4yourtype.com .

16-4. https://www.ncbi.nlm.nih.gov/pmc/articles/pmc1618732/.

17. EMOTIONAL STRESS

"The greatest weapon against stress is our
ability to choose one thought over another."
— *William James*

C ertainly dealing with arthritis can be emotionally
stressful; after all, you're in pain, and the longer you're
in pain, the more you're stressed. That can set up a
vicious cycle.

But what's also true is that emotional stress can contribute to
your arthritic state. In fact, because your emotional mind
influences your health all the time, including your arthritis, this
is already taking place even as you read this.

You may find it difficult to accept that with a symptom as
obviously physical as arthritis, you can harness your emotional
state in service of healing it. Think that's not true?

If you want to reap substantial healing dividends and more easily
free yourself from your arthritis, consider this: your internally-
held attitudes affect not just your physiology, they also
profoundly boost or diminish your ability to heal. How is this
possible?

This awareness has long been known and taught   references to
it exist in folk wisdom and in spiritual and esoteric teachings,
including ancient ones. To these are now added findings from a
variety of scientific disciplines that shed light on just how this
takes place.

Certain physiological truths are at work whether your emotional
state affects your symptoms positively or negatively. One of

these was demonstrated by Dr. Candace Pert, who confirmed that "thoughts become things". In other words, the thoughts you think –whether positive or negative - produce a physiological parallel.

Dr. Pert described these as 'molecules of the mind.' (17-1) These molecules begin to affect your physical state through your hypothalamus, a part of your brain that has wide control over a wide variety of cellular level functions.

"I've come to believe that virtually all illness, if not psychosomatic in foundation, has a definite psychosomatic component," she wrote. The "molecules of emotion," she argued, "run every system in our body," creating a "bodymind's intelligence" that is "wise enough to seek wellness" without a great deal of high-tech medical intervention. (17-2)

Dr. Bruce Lipton's work took this discovery further. He demonstrated how these molecules, once generated, interact with all your cell membranes. He revealed that your cell membranes are the actual 'brains' of your cells, constantly making 'choices' about what can enter inside the cell and what cannot. (17-3)

In other words, your cell membranes 'decide' which molecules to allow to enter inside your cells. That is how the molecules of your mind enter your cells and order them around. In fact, they even affect your DNA.

His groundbreaking research "revealed that genes were turned on and off, not by the genes themselves, but through external, environmental stimuli", which includes your mind molecules. These radical findings ran contrary to the long-held assumptions of genetic determinism and became one of the early heralds of an emerging scientific understanding called epigenetics.

This means your emotional brain gets not only the first but also the last word in affecting any physical outcome, including those programmed into your genetic code. Plus, this process takes place continually, regardless of the conscious desires of your logical brain.

This and other research gives scientific evidence for why affirmations, autogenous training, hypnosis and so forth can have such potent effects on your physical states.

To summarize what this means: your mindset - whether or not you're aware of it - becomes your physiology. The thoughts you generate are processed into the rest of your body by way of neurotransmitters to your nervous, endocrine, immune, and other systems. As such, they become biochemical events, turning your internally held attitudes into incredibly powerful directors of your internal physiology. And it also means you use this power to greatly enhance your capacity to heal, our next topic. (17-4)

ഴ

WHAT YOU CAN DO

How You Generate the 'Molecules of Your Mind' While ultimately all your thoughts are generated inside your own mind, there are also outside influences that encourage you to develop your mindset in certain directions. After all, contact with other people is an essential part of human life. Since before recorded history, people have always lived in groups. In fact, it's likely we would not have survived as a species if we had not had support from other humans. Clearly, relationships with others have survival value, both for each of us as individuals, and as a group.

Mind Molecules Generated from Outside Yourself. You, like all other humans, are also a social being, and as such, you're impacted by other people, circumstances and events. Even though you gain enormous survival value from human relationships, you can be pulled down by some of their disadvantages. No doubt you could compose quite a list of these if you decided to name them!

Of all the pressures you can experience from other people, the ones that have the greatest effect on your own mindset are the ones outside your own conscious awareness. Think of them like an 'emotional infection.'

An emotional infection is like a virus, only it's a 'mind molecule' generated by someone else and taken in by you. It's a feeling or experience one person disowns and handles by setting up another person (or people) or animal (!) to feel instead.

A classic example is someone who feels powerless from being chastised by a boss at work and comes home and kicks the dog. Another instance is the bully who disowns his or her own fear but sets up others to feel it instead by threatening them.

Sometimes in a family or organizational system, one person has this assigned role - to carry some disowned feeling or experience. That's likely never stated out loud as part of an agreement to marry, say, or as part of an employment contract. Instead it's communicated and enforced non-verbally, 'under the table'.

Take the example of an office assistant who compulsively arrives earlier than the boss and leaves later, having become 'emotionally infected' with the boss's fear of being abandoned. Without being aware of it, the assistant 'believes' at an emotional level that job security depends on protecting the boss from those feelings.

Freeing Yourself from 'Mind Molecules' from Outside Yourself

Step One, Awareness. Luckily, you can turn such circumstances into opportunities to grow and evolve. The first step to do so is to become aware of them. When you notice an emotion, you can ask yourself these simple questions:

> *"Whose feeling is this? Is it mine? Or someone else's that I'm carrying?"*

Step Two, Reflection. As you reflect on the answers that pop up, you may realize that the feeling or experience you're carrying belongs to your life partner or your boss or your child or your parent, and not to you. If you realize it belongs to you, take responsibility for it instead of passing it on to someone else.

A caution: Don't succumb to the temptation to pass the feeling back onto the person (or people or organization) from whom you got it. If you do that, you could spend the rest of your life struggling to get the other party to own it, and engaging in lots of arguments while doing so.

Step Three, Put it down. Instead, treat it as if you had just discovered you were holding some rotten, smelly bit of garbage. Instead of handing it to somebody else, *put it down*. You might even hold the image of an actual garbage can marked 'emotional refuse' and see yourself putting it in there.

Step Four, Notice What Happens. Then, awaken your thinking capacities. Next time you're in contact with that person or group or organization, notice what happens when invitations to pick up that disowned emotion get passed around, and you don't pick it up! Just watch – don't struggle or argue or get mad or in any way engage with it.

You'll find out just how much the stability of the other person/people/organization depended on your carrying it for them. You just might see the situation intensify briefly as the battle to get you to change your mind takes place.

Step Five, Watch Compassionately. This is the time to simply watch compassionately and practice staying strong - the pressure is only temporary, and you're back in a position of power over yourself. And you got there because you used this situation as an opportunity to become conscious - to grow and evolve. (17-5)

Mind Molecules Generated from Your Own Mind. Of course, not all 'molecules of your mind' originate outside yourself – some, perhaps even most, are generated in and by your own mind. Regardless of where they originate, once they become patterns or loops or deeply held convictions, they breed 'mind molecules', and those affect your physiology.

Arthritis Issues. The following are some emotional arenas that create 'mind molecules particularly relevant to arthritis in general:

- being able to move freely
- to be able to move forward
- to have freedom from feeling constrained
- to be safe to move, to release rather than hold anger
- to be flexible
- being able to move into the life you want
- confidence in being supported
- safely to release toxins

Infectious Arthritis. If you are dealing with parasites or viruses, you might find value in contemplating,

> *What person or situation in my life feels parasitic, like it's feeding off me?*
> Or, *What person or situation in my life is like a virus, getting inside my cells and bossing my DNA around, telling it what to do?*

> If your arthritis is connected to a toxic burden, consider, *What person or situation in my life is toxic to my physical and/or emotional wellbeing?*

Be assured that becoming aware of these stresses doesn't mean you'll suddenly have to quit your job, get a divorce, move away or any such thing. Instead, by awakening to what's stressing you, you'll be able to change your relationship to it, and in so doing, change the 'mind molecules' your body is delivering to your joints.

To assist you in discovering and releasing any mind patterns that may be contributing to your arthritis – or preventing you from healing it, the following are some resources you can use.

Resources to support using the healing power of your mind.
Now that you're aware of how mind molecules affect your body – especially your arthritis, you can make use of that ability to create 'mind molecules' that positively affect your symptoms and your healing process. In other words, you can begin to 'rewrite' relevant emotional attitudes.

One powerful way to do this is to listen to and take in healthy emotional messages, or 'emotional nutrients.'

That term may sound strange to you at first, but if you think about it a moment, you'll realize you've been taking in emotional messages all along – and further, that some of them nourish and sustain you and some are toxic and work against you. Being emotionally nourished creates the mind molecules that support your healing goals. (17-6)

If you are someone who didn't receive some key emotional nutrients that supported your healthy growth as you were growing up, you can find out what they are and take them in at *www.youremotionalnutrients.com.* Check out the free sample there, which you can click on and listen to any time.

If you would like guidance to upgrade your emotional life, you might benefit from the ebook: *Your Emotional Self, Five Secrets for a Successful Emotional Life* . (17-7)

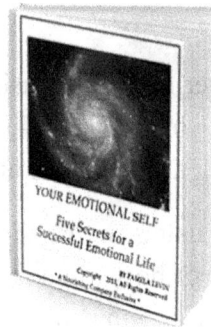

Figure 82 Summarizes the ingredients for a successful emotional life.
www.youremotionallife.com

No doubt your emotional state is one of the most powerful forces that can aid you (or defeat you!) in achieving the life you want, free from arthritis. Remember: you can harness its power because your emotional state - *whatever it is* - is processed into the rest of your body by way of neurotransmitters and your endocrine, immune and nervous systems.

SELF-HELP RESOURCES FOR EMOTIONAL STRESS

Tapping (Emotional Freedom Technique / EFT). Assists emotional heaping by tapping a sequence of Chinese acupressure points while focusing on an issue or stress and repeating a stress-related phrase. (17-8)

The Healing Code. Assists emotional healing to aid you in re-setting old thought patterns, beliefs and emotional charges. (17-9)

Trauma Release Exercise/ TRE. A series of exercises that assist the body in releasing deep muscular patterns of stress, tension and trauma. (17-10)

The above techniques represent a few of the many options available for self-healing of emotional trauma and stress. Using the above and the other resources described in these pages, you can direct that process in the service of becoming arthritis-free.

***

Endnotes

17-1. https://www.facebook.com/CandacePertLegacyPage.

17-2 Candace Pert, 67, *Explorerer of the Brain, Dies.* by John Schwartz NewYorkTimes.com Sept. 19, 2013. https://www.nytimes.com/2013/09/20/science/candace-pert-67-explorer-of-the-brain-dies.html

17-3. https://www.brucelipton.com/books/biology-of-belief.

17-4. http://www.betterhealthbytes.com/Volume-5-Issue-86.html.

17-5. http://www.betterhealthbytes.com/Volume-6-Issue-90.html.

17-6. http://www.youremotionalnutrients.com/.

17-7. http://www.youremotionallife.com/.

17-8. https://www.thetappingsolution.com/

17-9. See demonstrations here:
https://www.youtube.com/watch?v=xRGBlpOk82k
or https://www.youtube.com/watch?v=Y1Vk1fIODAk

17-10. https://www.youtube.com/watch?v=hTPFbd-5xmE

18. FINDING PROFESSIONAL HELP

"I learned to always take on things I'd never done before. Growth and comfort do not coexist."

Virginia Rometty (CEO of IBM)

B y now you've discovered that treatment of arthritis symptoms is very different than actually finding their causes and resolving them. That's been a key difference in the approach detailed in this book.

Also by now, you may be eager to get to the root of your own arthritis symptoms. You may remember from previous chapters how often you were advised to work with a health practitioner competent to find and address the various causes outlined here.

PHYSICAL HEALING RESOURCES

You will need to have reputable sources of whole food concentrates and herbs because that's what your body – *any* body- uses to heal and repair. You will also need the best and most reliable and well-trained health practitioner. To find both of these together, you'll want a licensed health practitioner who carries these remedies. And if you live outside the United States, you'll still need a U.S. practitioner to assess your situation and send you your protocol.

So, here's my best advice for finding the right one for you: look through the various contacts listed below and find names that cross-reference. For example, let's say you're looking for a good clinical nutritionist in your area. You might find some names of possible candidates near you through their professional association. Then, narrow that down to ones who are trained in clinical nutrition and the specific assessment methods that will reveal what your body needs to heal.

To find which ones on your list have that training and skill set, you might contact the training organizations listed below to find names of qualified professionals who've taken the trainings they offer. You can also check websites for any names you've uncovered.

You can follow the same procedure for any other licensed health professional, whether to assist you with your physical health or your emotional life.

And, of course, if you have a friend or relative who has experienced this approach and can make a recommendation to you, so much the better.

The bottom line is that these professionals exist all over – in small towns and large cities. So don't despair, the help you need is out there.

So here are the names of the various professional organizations, followed by the names of the training organizations.

Acupuncturists You can contact the American Association of Acupuncture and Oriental Medicine at https://www.aaaomonline.org/ They are the oldest and largest national membership organization of acupuncture and Oriental medicine (AOM) practitioners and supporters. Their purpose is to serve to advance the profession and practice of AOM.

Naturopathic Doctors To find a licensed naturopath in the US or Canada, contact the American Association of Naturopathic Physicians, https://www.naturopathic.org/ or the Canadian Naturopathic Association, https://www.cand.ca/findmynd/

Chiropractors To find a chiropractor who also does nutritional work, you can contact the American Chiropractic Association here: https://www.acatoday.org/Find-a-Doctor. Once you find some possible people in your area, check to see if they have a website, which will tell you what kind of work they do. If they use the words in the clinical training references below, you're in the right ballpark.

Nurses The American Holistic Nurses Association (AHNA) serves more than 4,600 members across the U.S., is the definitive voice for holistic nursing, and promotes the education of nurses, other healthcare professionals, and the public in all aspects of holistic caring and healing. http://www.ahna.org/

Homeopaths For information about homeopaths in North America, see the national center for homeopathy web site. http://www.homeopathycenter.org/

Clinical nutritionists: Clinical nutritionists are different than dieticians. Clinical nutritionists focus on identifying the specific nutrition your body needs to heal. You can contact them through their website: American Society for Clinical Nutrition. http://www.ascn.org/. Then cross-reference any names you receive with the training organizations listed below.

A heads-up before you do, however. The integrity of their _organization_ has been repeatedly called into question because of conflicts of interest with food companies which fund sessions at professional meetings and sponsor scientific studies in its professional journal. (18-1) Therefore, be sure to double check any names you uncover with the clinical training organizations listed below.

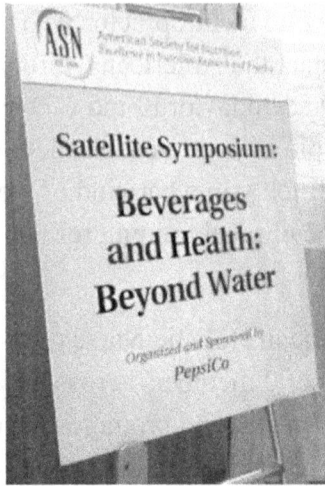

Figure 83 This 'professional' and 'scientific' meeting-about nutrition-has numerous corporate sponsors and influencers. This one is from PepsiCo.

Osteopaths Osteopaths are licensed to practice medicine in all US states, and use the initials D.O. (doctor of osteopathy) instead of M.D. Their website is here: http://www.osteopathic.org/pages/default.aspx.

Certified Herbalists: To find a health professional that specializes in herbs, you can check with the American Herbalists Guild, a non-profit, educational organization for the furtherance of herbalism. From there, you can check with the professional members whose names you receive to discover if they also have training in clinical nutrition, if they use whole food concentrates in their practice, if they have training in muscle testing, and if so what method (see below for recommended trainings.) Their contact is here: https://www.americanherbalistsguild.com.

Training Organizations: Throughout the U.S., there are representatives of Standard Process in various regions. They are the manufacturers of the organic whole food concentrates that are so potent in delivering health improvement results. They are also the exclusive US distributors of MediHerb, which manufacturers organic herbs guaranteed to contain the assorted medicinal constituents that make them clinically potent.

These SP representatives sponsor professional trainings in their areas and also have lists of licensed health professionals using their products. Do be aware, however, that having a Standard Process account is not the same as having the clinical training and competence to trace down the origins of your arthritic symptoms. Thus heed the advice to cross-reference, especially with the organization recommendations from the other training organizations below.

That said, you can go to the Standard Process website. They are makers of the powerful whole food concentrates and whole organic herbs. Find the name of the representatives in your area. Contact them through the emails or office numbers listed there. When you do, request a referral to a practitioner whom they know is good with finding and addressing *causes* of arthritis. Contact them at www.StandardProcess.com

Training Organization for **Nutrition Response Testing is a** professional training organization developed by chiropractor Freddie Ulan. His organization sends qualified trainers to every corner of the United States. His methods are ones I continue to use in my own practice, and I highly recommend them. They may be able to give you the names of some graduates in your area. Their contact information is: Ulan Nutritional Systems, Inc., http://www.unsinc.info/nutrition-response-testing.html.

Their own definition is: "Nutrition Response Testing is a non-invasive system of analyzing the body in order to determine the underlying causes of ill health. When these are corrected through safe, natural, nutritional means, the body can repair itself in order to attain and maintain more optimum health." Contact them at Nutrition Response Testing - Ulan Nutritional Systems www.unsinc.info/nutrition-response-testing.html

You can also check out some YouTube videos to get a better idea of what you might expect. You might start with: *Nutrition Response Testing - What to Expect on the First Visit* – YouTube Video for Nutrition Response Testing https://www.youtube.com/watch?v=eYb6_w5nusc

***Training Organization for* Morphogenetic Field Technique** offers professional training throughout the United States by its founder, Frank Springob, D.C.. He is a chiropractic physician, author and educator, and is the co-developer with Autumn Smith, NTP of Morphogenic Field Technique (MFT).

This is their description, "Morphogenic Field Technique is an innovative energy signature testing procedure for homeopathic, nutritional and herbal practitioners who want to do more for their patients. It originates ("genic") positive change ("morph") and harnesses the power of the body's energy fields at the cellular level. It is an integrated holistic approach that involves 100% natural and nutritional protocols custom matched to each individual's needs."

This is a cutting edge healing method based on quantum physics, totally non-invasive. I place a high value on this way of assessing and recommending treatment protocols. You can contact them through their website, http://morphogenicfieldtechnique.com. While there, you can also access videos that demonstrate how MFT works.

Make a list of organizations you'd like to contact. Once you do, narrow that list to people in your area.

When you have some key names and are ready to contact them, prepare yourself with a list of questions.
Some of these will be unique to you, but you may want to include the following:

1. Do you do NRT (Nutrition Response Testing).
2 .Do you do MFT (Morphogenetic Field Testing).
3. Do you use Standard Process whole food supplements
    and/or MediHerb products?
4. What is your training in any of the above?

Once you make a choice and experience that practitioner, check in with your gut to see how you feel. You can't necessarily gauge that choice on how quickly you get results, because your body and its healing process is on nature's timetable, and no one, including the best practitioner in the world, can change that.

EMOTIONAL LIFE RESOURCES

If you sense your emotional life would benefit from greater emotional intelligence, so your stress level becomes lower at work and in your relationships, consider taking advantage of seven free, short mini-course lessons to raise your emotional intelligence. (18-2)

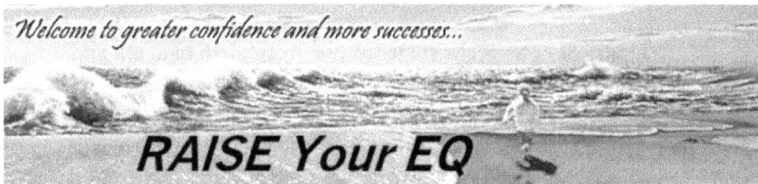

Welcome to greater confidence and more successes...

RAISE Your EQ

**Figure 84 A free mini-course to raise your
emotional intelligence at www.raiseeq.com**

If you feel you need a map of the entire emotional landscape, check out emotional development 101, available at www.emotionaldevelopment101.com. (18-3)

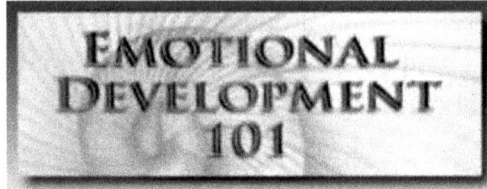

Figure 85 Life's emotional landscape from your first through last breath, along with how to navigate it emotionally.

For a book that covers all the emotional stages of life from first breath through the last, get a copy of *Cycles of Power, a User's Guide to the Seven Seasons of Life.* (18-4)

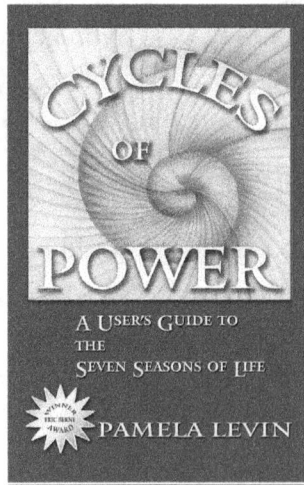

Figure 86 The cyclic stages of life from birth to death and how to grow in healthy ways in each of its stages.

Last, to reduce your stress, and even possibly your arthritic pain, consider tapping, or EFT (emotional freedom technique). There are short videos on YouTube that show you how to do this technique yourself. Since people who try it out are often amazed by the positive results they receive, you may want to try it several times and find out for yourself.

Don't turn yourself into a gerbil on a wheel, going round and round and not getting anywhere. Instead, review this section.

CONCLUSION

Now you know not only the wide range of causes that can underlie one symptom, you also have the empowering information you need to deal with each one. Together, you can use these to free yourself from debilitating pain and live the life of your dreams.

***

Endnotes:

18-1. https://www.foodpolitics.com/2013/11 /conflicts-of-interest-in-nutrition-societies-american-society-of-nutrition/

18-2. http://raiseeq.com.

18-3. http://www.emotionaldevelopment101.com.

18-4. https://www.amazon.com/Cycles-Power-Pamela-Levin/dp/0967271819.

INDEX OF IMAGE SOURCES

Image on flyleaf from https://loudounsportstherapy
com/wp-content/uploads/2013/08/Arthritis-2-1.jpg \

Figure 1. https://userscontent2.emaze.com/images/
2a4ce32f-1824-424e-9dd8-ebcb61acb1f1/
85dbb9e167a893a62deb6ebbd7305c52.jpg.

Figure 2. http://www.sheffieldphysiotherapy.
co.uk/wp-content/uploads/2017/08/joint-pain-elbow-arthritis.jpg.

Figure 3. http://www.stanfordchildrens.org/en/
topic/default?id=anatomy-of-a-joint-85-P00044.

Figure 4. https://www.fda.gov/ucm/groups/fdagov-
public/documents/image/ucm453626.png.

Figure 5. https://i.ytimg.com/vi/Vspb3bi_uV4/
hqdefault.jpg.

Figure 6. http://static.panoramio.com/photos/large/
11871446.jpg.

Figure 7. https://encryptedbn0.gstatic.com/images?
q=tbn:ANd9GcTYPDwUwVqTZFDnAWm_Ivjep-
1V1_nOlOXLY2qJ6760KjVIzaVJ.

Figure 8. http://lewisandclark.today/1804_8/images/
wild_black_currant_101.jpg.

Figure 9. http://blog.growingwithscience.com/wp-
content/uploads/2012/07/moth-evening-primrose.jpg.

Figure 10. https://upload.wikimedia.org/wikipedia/
commons/thumb/4/4c/pikutanni-test.jpg/330px-
Epikutanni-test.jpg.

Figure 11. https://cdn.pixabay.com/photo/2016/05/26/18/18/cereals-1417868__340.jpg.

Figure 12. http://glutenfreewithjudee.blogspot.com/2017/08/low-carb-japanese-eggplant-grill-t-side.html.

Figure 13. https://encrypted-tbn0.gstatic.com/images?q=tbn:ANd9GcSXgddQZwrLf5Gmg9iUpwL_jE9ts6I0lgO0KlIVVq7E_CMHDr_8DQ.

Figure 14. https://sc01.alicdn.com/kf/UT88p1uXEJXXXagOFbXz/Fresh-tomatoes.jpg.

Figure 15. https://blog.oxforddictionaries.com/wp-content/uploads/potato.jpg.

Figure 16. https://paulaowens.com/wp-content/uploads/2014/04/metals9.jpg .

Figure 17. http://www.sott.net/image/s14/281721/full/are_you_doing_the_right_things.jpg.

Figure 18. http://www.preventivemedicalcenteromarin.com/wp-content/uploads/2015/07/doctrdataurineref.jpg.

Figure 19. http://www.freeoftoxicmetals.com/Your-Toxic-Metal-Burden-Book.html.

Figure 20. http://www.trustedhealthproducts.com/blog/wp-content/uploads/2015/03/synthetic-chemicals.jpg.

Figure 21. https://response.restoration.noaa.gov/sites/default/files/images/13/dolphin-dead-on-beach-staff-records-data_credit-lousiana-dept-fisheries-wildlife_356_0.jpg.

Figure 22. https://3c1703fe8d.site.internapcdn.net /newman/gfx/news/hires/2017/syntheticche.jpg.

Figure 23. https://s-media-cache-ak0.pinimg.com/ originals/ab/57/94/ab5794040220b4cbc3231 ff85fea6821.jpg.

Figure 24. https://www.capcvet.org/maps#2017/all/lyme-disease/dog/united-states/.
Figure 25. http://lymediseaseuk.com/wp-content/uploads/2013/10/zd-ticks-onfinger.jpg.

Figure 26. http://lymediseaseuk.com/2016/02/10/tick-bite-prevention-and-removal/.

Figure 27. https://www.cdc.gov/lyme/images/rashes/ CDC_EM.jpg.

Figure 28. https://previews.123rf.com/images/ jarun011/jarun0111706/jarun011170600086/ 80250154-strongyloides-stercoralis-in-stool-analyze-by-microscope.jpg.

Figure 29. https://commons.wikimedia.org/w/ index.php?curid=36876126.

Figure 30. https://www.cdc.gov/parasites/hipworm/index.

Figure 31. Ibid.

Figure 32. http://www.scienceagogo.com/ news/img/flu_virus.jpg.

Figure 33. https://www.std-gov.org/images/Hepatitis-C-2-640x600.jpg.

Figure 34. .https://i2.wp.com/www.medicalook.com/ diseases_images/hepatitis-b.jpg.

Figure 35. https://upload.wikimedia.org/wikipedia/
commons/4/4e/Peelbark_St._Johns-wort_%28
Hypericum_fasciculatum%29_%286439017119%29.jpg.

Figure 36. https://bluestoneperennials.global.ssl.
astly.net/img/ecpu/650/ecpu_0_echinacea_
purpurea.1491333866.jpg.

Figure 37. https://nccih.nih.gov/sites/nccam.nih.gov
/files/herbs/astragalus.jpg.

Figure 38. https://cdn-images-1.medium.com/max/
523/1*ZA8Ng7T72zaQNEkEcR0JBw.png.

Figure 39. http://www.onegreenplanet.org/vegan-food/sesame-
seeds-health-benefits-tips-and-recipes/.
Figure 40. http://www.healthplusinc.com/uploads/9/0/
5/8/90584463/burdock-root-product-ingredient-for-super-blood-
every-day-cleanse-vineveracosmetics_2.png.

Figure 41. https://upload.wikimedia.org/wikipedia/
commons/thumb/d/d3/staphylococcus_aureus_visa _2.jpg/220px-
staphylococcus_aureus_visa_2.jpg.

Figure 42. https://www.cdc.gov/media/subtopic/
library/DiseaseAgents/img35.jpg.
Figure 43. http://images.medicaldaily.com/sites/
medicaldaily.com/files/2014/08/26/gonorrhea-
bacterium.jpg .

Figure 44. http://a360-wp-ploads.s3.amazonaws.com/
wp-content/uploads/rtmagazi/2014/04/bacteria-500-
466x298.jpg.

Figure 45. https://breadcakesandale.files.wordpress.com /2014/03/unproved.jpg?w=768&h=510.

Figure 46. Ibid.

Figure 47. http://faculty.ccbcmd.edu/courses/bio141/ lecguide/unit4/fungi/images/candida.jpg.

Figure 48. https://www.nationalcandidacenter.com/ Self-Test-2-My-Body-Fluids-s/1877.htm.

Figure 49. Licensed under the creative commons attribution-share alike 3.0 unported license.

Figure 50. http://www.blackmoldmildewremoval. com/wp-content/uploads/Strachybotrys-Blackold.jpg.

Figure 51. Ibid.

Figure 52. Image courtesy: US National Library of Medicine. Image source: ottman n, smidt h, de vos wm and belzer c (2012) the function of our microbiota: who is out there and what do they do? Front. Cell. Inf. Microbio. 2:104. Doi: 10.3389/fcimb.2012.00104.

Figure 53. http://www.flspinalcord.us/what-is-peyers-patches/what-is-peyers-patches-the-peyers-patches-anatomy-of-the-peyers-patches-anatomy/

Figure 54. http://i2.cdn.cnn.com/cnnnext/dam/assets/ 130128114946-gluten-intestine-damagae-horizontal-large-gallery.jpg.

Figure 55. http://azchironeuro.com/wp-content/ uploads/2017/05/dr-axe-leaky-gut-278x300.jpg.

Figure 56. https://www.viome.com.

Figure 57. https://dnfitness.files.wordpress.com/2014/01/phscale.jpg.

Figure 58. http://altered-states.net/barry/update178/DigestiveTract.jpg.

Figure 59. https://sites.google.com/a/richland2.org/cameron-diamond-amyah-ph-project/_/rsrc/1461176730208/home/the-ph/My%20Ph%20Scale.jpg.

Figure 60. http://3.bp.blogspot.com/-f4bO-rNHBs/VKhZjaJ2kkI/AAAA AAAA00E/4lcpW7Qik2s/s1600/AppleCiderVinegar_www.hypo global.com.jpg.

Figure 61. http://www.moondragon.org/health/disorders/arthritis.html.

Figure 62. Ibid.

Figure 63. http://ard.bmj.com/content/58/5/261.

Figure 64. http://ard.bmj.com/content/ann rheumdis/58/5/261/f1.large.jpg.

Figure 65. http://media1.s-nbcnews.com/i/msnbc/Components/Interactives/Health/MiscHealth/GOUT.gif.

Figure 66. http://www.web-books.com/eLibrary/Medicine/Physiology/Skeletal/Joint.htm.

Figure 67. https://www.southerncross.co.nz/-/media/images/medical-library/osteoarthritis-1.jpg. (Graphic courtesy of A. Bonsall and edicineNet.com).

Figure 68. http://www.oilsfats.org.nz/wp-content/uploads/2014/02/OliveOils-670.jpg.

Figure 69. https://montereybayholistic.files.
wordpress.com/2014/08/hemp-seed-oil1.jpg.

Figure 70. https://img.wikinut.com/img/qguyukoc
7xz9ncoj/jpeg/0/cis-and-trans-fats.jpeg.

Figure 71. https://goldfieldsosteopathy.files.
wordpress.com/2013/12/poustie_15122013_
0167-edit-edit.jpg.

Figure 72. https://www.researchgate.net/figure/
283159577_figure-2-anthropometric-data-collection-form.

Figure 73. https://ohsonline.com/articles/2014/09/01/
~/media/images/2014/09/914paulausky1.jpg.
Figure 74 http://www.birdcronin.com/pains/images/
tennis_elbow.jpg.

Figure 75. http://sci.washington.edu/info/forums/
reports/shoulder_health.asp.

Figure 76. http://www.medrego.com/wp-
content/uploads/2017/11/tissue-healing-eng-1-300x229.jpg.

Figure 77. www. studentconsult.com

Figure 78. http://www.holistic-healing-
information.com/images/jointpainauto3.jpg.

Figure 79. http://images.wisegeek.com/diagram-depicting-
rheumatoid-arthritis.jpg.

Figure 80. https://en.wikipedia.org/wiki/file:
phytohemagglutinin_l.png.

Figure 81. https://www.mdidea.com/products/
new/r086/rehmanniarootwithleaves.jpg.

Figure 82. http:// www.youremotionallife.com.

Figure 83. http://www.raiseeq.com.

Figure 84. http://www.emotionaldevelopment101.com

Figure 85. http:// http://yourcycleoflife.com/cycles-of-power.htm.

Figure 86. https://www.foodpolitics.com/wp-content/uploads/Picture12-210x300.jpg

***

ABOUT PAMELA LEVIN

I founded the ***Nourishing Company*** with the motivation to provide practical information to *"nourish body, mind and spirit so you and your relationships can thrive."* This book continues that intention by offering empowering information for improving your health.

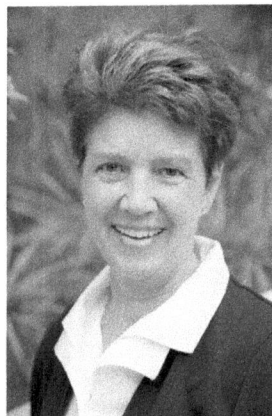

I began learning effective ways to do that first in the medical/hospital setting, then in the emotional realm, and now in clinical nutrition and herbology.

I'm passionate about sharing what I've learned so others can gain the health victories they need. That's why I continue to publish what I learn.

I'm 75 now, and when I'm not seeing clients or writing, I enjoy hiking, swimming, gardening, yoga, playing with my grandchildren and making music with friends.

OTHER PUBLICATIONS BY PAMELA LEVIN

Books:

Perfect Bones: A Six-Point Plan for Healthy Bones

The Female Hormone Journey: Lifetime Care of Your Hormones

Your Emotional Self: Five Secrets for a Successful Emotional Life

Your Toxic Metal Burden: How to Safely Lighten Your Load

The Cycle of Life: Creating Smooth Passages in Every Life Season

Cycles of Power: A User's Guide to the Seven Seasons of Life

Online programs:

Emotional Development 101

Your Emotional Nutrients

Natural Female Hormone Care

Raise Your EQ

Newsletter:

Betterhealthbytes.com

Award:

The International Transactional Analysis Association's prestigious Eric Berne Scientific Award

Access her award speech here: http://nourishingcompany.com/pdf/eric-berne-speech.pdf.